T0192947

Hospitals and Community Benefit: New Demands, New Approaches

Your board, staff, or clients may also benefit from this book's insight. For more information on quantity discounts, contact the Health Administration Press Marketing Manager at (312) 424–9470.

This publication is intended to provide accurate and authoritative information in regard to the subject matter covered. It is sold, or otherwise provided, with the understanding that the publisher is not engaged in rendering professional services. If professional advice or other expert assistance is required, the services of a competent professional should be sought.

The statements and opinions contained in this book are strictly those of the authors and do not represent the official positions of the American College of Healthcare Executives or the Foundation of the American College of Healthcare Executives.

Reprinted August 2017

Library of Congress Cataloging-in-Publication Data

Evashwick, Connie J.
  Hospitals and community benefit : new demands, new approaches / Connie J. Evashwick.
    pages cm
  Includes bibliographical references.
  ISBN 978-1-56793-592-9 (alk. paper)
  1. Hospital and community. 2. Community health services. 3. Health services administration. I. Title.
  RA965.5.E93 2013
  362.11–dc23
                        2012051091

The paper used in this publication meets the minimum requirements of American National Standard for Information Sciences—Permanence of Paper for Printed Library Materials, ANSI Z39.48-1984. ∞ ™

Acquisitions editor: Janet Davis; Project manager: Amy Carlton; Cover designer: Marisa Jackson; Layout: Virginia Byrne

Found an error or a typo? We want to know! Please e-mail it to hapbooks@ache.org, and put "Book Error" in the subject line.

For photocopying and copyright information, please contact Copyright Clearance Center at www.copyright.com or at (978) 750–8400.

Health Administration Press
A division of the Foundation of the American
    College of Healthcare Executives
One North Franklin Street, Suite 1700
Chicago, IL 60606–3529
(312) 424–2800

Foreword

Recently I was in Nakuru, Kenya, working with the Presbyterian Church of East Africa Nakuru West on a project to expand a health clinic. It was Women's Guild Sunday, and the ladies were collecting a special offering for the clinic. This congregation is made up of people from the poorest areas of Nakuru who are dedicated to serving their neighbors. The call to help the clinic was urgent, as it was in serious need of funds to upgrade services. Despite their limited means, members of the church's congregation raised 470,000 Kenyan shillings, or approximately $6,000—which is a small fortune in Kenya. I was amazed! I asked one of the ladies, "How is this possible?" She replied, "Oh, you need to understand—we love with all our hearts."

That was such an incredible reminder of the power of love for the community as we in the hospital field struggle with limited resources to serve the health needs of the United States. There may be no better indicator of a US hospital's love for its community than in the community benefit (CB) programs it offers. Certainly, US hospitals have been providing remarkable community services, and the new mandates from the Internal Revenue Service and the Patient Protection and Affordable Care Act will result in expanding these yet further.

Hospitals and Community Benefit: New Demands, New Approaches is a well-researched, practical guide for hospitals striving to enhance the value of their CB programs and seeking to ensure compliance with external regulatory requirements. Hospitals have always been engaged with their communities in one way or another. This work by Connie Evashwick challenges us to manage community programs more effectively and provides helpful how-to's.

The US healthcare system continues to wrestle with how to develop, execute, and measure the impact of community-oriented programs most effectively. The rigor that is routinely brought to bear on other areas of hospital operations is too often not apparent in the operation of CB programs and related activities. This book addresses these concerns directly.

The love for community that underpins the hospital executive's profession demands that we go beyond regulatory compliance in the delivery of CB programs. The American College of Healthcare Executives' Policy Statement on Healthcare Executives' Responsibility to their Communities (Appendix) was first passed in 1989, and it continues to be renewed and reaffirmed. We must press to achieve the highest possible "return on investment" for the resources that are dedicated to community programs. Our constituencies deserve nothing less than the full measure of the organization's management competence.

I am impressed that this book provides both the explanation of what needs to be done and practical recommendations on how to do it. This new resource is important as a reference at the C-suite level and for directors of CB programs. It is also a helpful guide in ensuring that the board is up to date regarding the regulatory expectations for CB programs, needs assessments, and improvement plans. The reader will come away from this book with a much better understanding of what is required and, more important, what can be done to make programs for the community even more valu-able to the institution and to the people it serves.

Charles R. Evans, FACHE
President/CEO
International Health Services Group
Alpharetta, Georgia

Preface

Hospitals have been an integral component of community life since they began; serving the community is the essence of a hospital's mission. However, over the past few years, external pressures have brought new legal mandates accompanied by changes in community expectations. The Patient Protection and Affordable Care Act (ACA), the Internal Revenue Service (IRS), and tax regulations of a number of states all require a reexamination of the role of the hospital and other healthcare providers in relation to the community. The purposes of this book are:

- to advise healthcare leaders of the latest trends and regulatory obligations of hospitals with regard to the community, particularly with respect to the IRS and ACA;

- to highlight the bodies of information that can be used to pursue an evidence-based approach to activities in the community;
- to identify community partners and activities appropriate for collaboration, particularly in light of the ACA; and
- to recommend specific actions to ensure a hospital's viability within the context of current community expectations.

This book is written for executives and trustees of hospitals because hospitals are the institution of focus for the IRS and many of the ACA initiatives. However, the implications are relevant to those leading all types of healthcare organizations because the new measures have changed what communities expect from their partners in healthcare.

—*Connie J. Evashwick*

Acknowledgments

I would like to thank those who reviewed drafts of this book: Eileen Barsi, Michael Bilton, Charles Evans, Robert Sigmond, and Dr. Lawrence Weiss. I appreciate their dedication to the accuracy of the written document as well as their respective commitments to excellence in the broad field of hospital–community relations. The Association for Community Health Improvement and the Catholic Health Association's Community Benefit program both deserve recognition for promoting the complex work of hospital–community interactions.

CHAPTER 1

The New Imperative for Engagement

The role of the hospital in the community has been articulated, examined, and reexamined over the years. What has changed? The premise of this book is that in the context of health reform in the United States, healthcare organizations—and hospitals specifically—must be engaged with their communities in deliberate ways with measurable outcomes of their contributions. In today's environment, a hospital's success in strategic positioning, financing, marketing, and efficiency of operations all depend on engagement with the community. In addition to strategic benefits, the Internal Revenue Service (IRS) and the Patient Protection and Affordable Care Act (ACA) have created specific legal and financial reasons for hospitals to work closely with their communities. Moreover, hospital interaction with the community must be measurable—what is done, how many people are served, how many dollars are involved, and ultimately, what the impact of the hospital is on the health of the community. What is new is not the hospital's commitment to its community; it is the prescription of what must be done and how.

HISTORY AND EVOLUTION

Historically, hospitals grew from community need. The history of the hospital, both internationally and in the United States, is well documented. The mission statement of many hospitals includes explicit reference to the community (see Exhibit 1.1). Benjamin Franklin and colleague Dr. Thomas Bond established Pennsylvania Hospital in Philadelphia in 1751 as the nation's first hospital supported by action of the state legislature. The cornerstone, written by Franklin, reads (University of Pennsylvania Health System 2012):

In the year of Christ
MDCCLV.
George the second happily reigning
(for he sought the happiness of his people)

Philadelphia flourishing
(for its inhabitants were publick spirited)
this building
by the bounty of the government,
and of many private persons,
was piously founded
for the relief of the sick and miserable;
may the God of mercies
bless this undertaking.

Meeting the needs of the community has been the basis for hospitals in the United States across centuries and across the nation.

The American College of Healthcare Executives (ACHE) and the American Hospital Association (AHA) as well as other groups, such as the Catholic Health Association (CHA) and VHA, Inc., have sponsored various initiatives over the years to demonstrate, promote, and document the contributions of the hospital to the community. The AHA sponsors, through the Hospital Research and Educational Trust, the affiliate Association for Community Health Improvement (ACHI); membership in this organization includes individuals who work at the intersection of hospitals and communities (ACHI 2012). The AHA also launched Community Connections, which annually produces a compilation of hospital best practices with their communities (AHA 2012a). CHA created its Social Accountabil-

EXHIBIT 1.1 Sample Mission Statements
(Italics added for emphasis)

Sibley Memorial Hospital

Sibley Memorial is a community hospital offering healthcare services to people living in the Washington, DC, area.

Mission Statement

The mission of Sibley Memorial Hospital is to provide quality health services and facilities for *the community*, to promote wellness, to relieve suffering, and to restore health as swiftly, safely, and humanely as it can be done, consistent with the best service we can give at the highest value for all concerned.

St. Joseph's Hospital and Medical Center

A member of Dignity Health, St. Joseph's Medical Center is a comprehensive health system based in Phoenix, Arizona, that includes four hospitals, clinics, imaging centers, physician groups, an insurance company, and a strong community outreach program.

Mission, Vision, and Values: Dignity Health and St. Joseph's Hospital and Medical Center are committed to furthering the healing ministry of Jesus, and to providing high-quality, affordable healthcare to *the communities* we serve.

Our Mission

Dignity Health and our Sponsoring Congregations are committed to furthering the healing ministry of Jesus. We dedicate our resources to:

- Delivering compassionate, high-quality, affordable health services;
- Serving and advocating for our sisters and brothers who are poor and disenfranchised; and
- *Partnering with others in the community* to improve the quality of life.

Pennsylvania Hospital

Pennsylvania Hospital provides diagnostic and therapeutic medical services to the residents of Philadelphia. As part of the University of Pennsylvania Health System, it also serves as a teaching and clinical research institution.

Mission Statement

We believe that Pennsylvania Hospital, the nation's first hospital, has a responsibility to:

- Ensure access to superior quality integrated health care for *our community* and expand access for underserved populations within *the community*
- Create a supportive team environment for patients, employees, and clinical staff
- Foster learning and growth through comprehensive academic and educational relationships
- Exhibit stewardship and creativity in the management of all available resources

SOURCES: Sibley Memorial Hospital (2012); St. Joseph's Hospital and Medical Center (2012); Pennsylvania Hospital (2012).

ity program in the late 1980s and today maintains an active program of information, publications, and conferences for those engaged in community benefit (CHA 1989, 2012b).

Weil, Bogue, and Morton (2001) conducted a study on behalf of AHA and ACHE to determine best practices among hospitals recognized for modeling leadership in working with their communities. Despite the array of hospital–community interactions, the authors state, "not-for-profits derive their legitimacy and social support from the perception that they are working to meet community needs. . . . But no commonly recognized practices exist to ensure that hospitals hold themselves accountable to serve their community." This lack of accountability led ultimately to the enactment of specific and stringent reporting imposed by the IRS starting in 2008 but rolling out through 2014. In its efforts to expand access to healthcare services, the ACA placed further responsibilities on the hospital. Thus, what is new is the stringent accountability for community involvement that hospital senior executives must understand and implement.

EXTERNAL PRESSURES

Strategically, hospitals must be responsive to the community to accomplish business goals. The old adage about "doing good to do well" holds more than ever before. Over the past 40 years, hospitals have experienced the ups and downs of radically changing markets, myriad external pressures, and business innovations that took off wildly then failed dismally. Today's legal and regulatory climate mandates involvement with the community in specific ways, as described later in this chapter. But even beyond regulatory compliance, understanding one's community will be essential for success in business operations (Evashwick and Barsi 2012). Evolutions in public health practice, communications technology, and consumer choice all reinforce the importance of community involvement for market positioning and strategic directions. Managing chronic illness, assuming responsibility for population segments through accountable care organizations (ACOs), handling an expanded Medicaid population efficiently—all these benefit from a public health, or community, perspective on evidence-based healthcare man-

EXHIBIT 1.2 External Pressures and Trends Leading to Collaboration with the Community

External Pressures and Trends	Collaborators	Collaborative Efforts
Community health needs assessments	Local public health experts	Inclusion mandated by ACA
Accountable care organizations	Physicians and insurers	Patient-centered medical homes
Internal Revenue Service	Community organizations	Activities defined by Schedule H
Electronic health record exchanges	Healthcare providers	RHIOs, EHR
Population health focus	Public health departments	Health promotion
Global spread of infectious diseases	Public health departments	Surveillance
Domination of chronic diseases	Physicians and LTC orgs	Continuity of care
Social media	Lay population	Electronic information exchange
Aging population	Long-term care providers	Patient transfer agreements
Renewed emphasis on prevention	Physicians and clinics	Communitywide prevention
Emergency response readiness	Gov't and private organizations	Emergency plans
Wellness initiatives	Employers	Employee wellness programs
Medicaid expansion, prevention	Insurers, managed care	Recruitment and utilization programs

agement. In suggesting the "Pillars of Excellence" that a healthcare organization use as a basis for its management framework, the six-pillar Studer Group model lists community of equal importance with financing and strategic planning (Studer 2009). Exhibit 1.2 highlights some of the many external pressures creating a renaissance in hospital–community collaboration.

ACTIONS FOR LEADERSHIP

What can hospital executives do to work with the community to meet legal and regulatory requirements as well as optimize marketing and business strategies? Consider the actions taken by those healthcare institutions that have been leaders in community engagement: understanding the significance of the community, making performance with the community evidence-based and measurable, and communicating with stakeholders. Weil, Bogue, and Reed (2001) offered model structures and processes derived from analyzing high-performing institutions, as did the program *Advancing the State of the Art in Community Benefit* (Public Health Institute 2004).

Dignity Health recognized the importance of being accountable for the health of the community several years ago. The system includes the improvement of community health status as one of the evaluation criteria for its CEOs, a clear message about the importance of community involvement with a precise measure to be monitored and reported to the board (Barsi 2009). Catholic health organizations realized that their contributions to their communities were often overlooked or not understood. The Social Accountability project developed an elaborate system to document and report organizations' activities to foster a healthy community (CHA 1989). CHA sponsored the creation of an accounting format called CBISA, the Community Benefit Inventory for Social Accountability, which today has been adopted by

many hospitals beyond Catholic institutions (Lyon Software 2012). Reporting to stakeholders and celebrating communitywide success has become standard practice for many hospitals, such as those that have applied for the AHA's Foster G. McGaw Prize for Excellence in Community Service or the Jackson Healthcare National Hospital Charitable Service Award (AHA 2012b; Jackson Healthcare 2013).

In short, achieving effective community engagement is not a mystery. Doing it requires the commitment of senior healthcare executives and board members based on a solid understanding of legal mandates, effective techniques, and, perhaps most important, the community.

PURPOSE OF THE BOOK

The purpose of this book is to walk busy healthcare executives through current mandates and contemporary practices of successful hospital–community relationships. Healthcare executives will recognize that the management principles are not new—but an awareness of the need to apply good management to issues outside and within the walls of the hospital is essential. Readers should come away with ideas for governance, infrastructure, operations, collaboration, and measurement. Each can be used to maximize successful relationships with the community.

ACTIONS FOR HEALTHCARE EXECUTIVES

- Be aware of recent legal and regulatory changes that govern hospital relationships with the community and the implications of those changes for hospital policies and practices.
- Reevaluate how the hospital's strategic directions affect and are affected by the community at large and community leaders in particular.
- Embark on an initiative to revisit how the hospital structures, funds, measures, and reports its engagement with the community.

CHAPTER 2

Community Health: A Measurable Management Task

O ne challenge to community engagement is that it can be perceived as a "soft" activity, with amorphous borders and no measurable outcomes. This is not the case. To appreciate why hospitals must pay attention to the community and to know how to do so effectively, hospital leaders must understand how community health is conducted today and how it can be used to help accomplish the hospital's mission. An evidence-based approach to management is as applicable to community health as it is to any of the other management tasks of the hospital. The relationship of community health to the formal discipline of public health is particularly important.

DEFINITIONS

Community benefit (CB) is a term used by the Internal Revenue Service (IRS) to refer to specific actions that allow a nonprofit hospital to maintain its tax exemption (IRS 2012a). This term is discussed in detail in Chapter 3. This book uses CB with this specific definition rather than as a generic term.

Community health is an amorphous concept and a term whose meaning lacks consensus. This lack of clarity is made worse by the IRS allowing each hospital to define its own community and indeed to declare that it serves several communities. For the purposes of this book, we will refer to *community health* as measurable by indicators of community health status and *community health activities* as those activities intended to improve the health of the community on a discrete and measurable dimension. A hospital might serve multiple communities, some of which are the focus of its formal CB activities while others are served for its mission without regard to IRS reporting or tax consequences. In using the term *community health*, the community of reference should be made explicit, not assumed.

Public health is a broad and potentially all-encompassing field of practice, as well as academic discipline. It is defined by the Institute of Medicine (2002) as "any activities undertaken to improve the health and well-being of the greater community." It places a great emphasis on prevention of healthcare problems. The Centers for Disease Control and Prevention (CDC 2012a) has identified ten essential public health functions—the practical tasks done by government public health departments (see Exhibit 2.1). These same functions are the basis for the new accreditation available to local and state health departments through the Public Health Accreditation Board (PHAB 2012). As an academic discipline, public health is taught in schools of public health, medicine, nursing, and other health professions universities as well as in burgeoning undergraduate programs offered by liberal arts colleges. Academic graduate training in public health typically includes the subjects of epidemiology, biostatistics, behavioral health, environmental health, and health management and policy. Some would argue that nutrition is also a core element of public health.

EXHIBIT 2.1 Ten Essential Public Health Functions

1. Monitor health status to identify community problems.

2. Diagnose and investigate health problems and hazards.

3. Inform, educate, and empower people about health issues.

4. Mobilize community partnerships.

5. Develop policies and plans.

6. Enforce laws and regulations.

7. Provide personal healthcare services when unavailable.

8. Ensure a competent public and personal health workforce.

9. Evaluate effectiveness, accessibility, and quality.

10. Research innovative solutions to health problems.

SOURCE: CDC (2012a).

Population health is another general term with multiple interpretations. It is "used to describe different strategies that can be developed and implemented to improve health and the quality of care while also managing costs" (McAlearney 2003). Population health overlaps with public health but has different connotations. The term is a bit of a misnomer in that it is applied to programs that target segments of the population rather than the entire population. Physicians and the medical profession use the term to refer to how disease states are approached on a populationwide rather than on an individual patient level.

Hospitals, like physicians, have realized that treating individual patients alone cannot prevent communitywide disasters. Preventing a negative occurrence at a community level is more cost-effective for the hospital than having one occur for which the hospital loses money on dozens or even hundreds of individual patients. The cost–benefit of preventing a negative health occurrence rather than remediating it is clear in many instances, but some elusive conditions avoid measurement. The challenge is often to persuade a single institution, such as a hospital, that investing in a population-wide activity, such as vaccination, that reaches many individuals beyond its own patients is in its best financial interest. Activities for which the cause-and-effect has not been demonstrated incontrovertibly or those with a long time lag between action and impact present similar challenges. Board commitment and an understanding of public and population health are essential in these situations.

EPIDEMIOLOGY 101

Epidemiology is the best example of the intersection of public health and population health—and their relevance to the hospital. Modern epidemiology was propelled by Dr. John Snow's 1854 discovery that the incidence of fatalities from a London cholera epidemic congregated around the water pump at Broad Street. The science of epidemiology has now advanced to employ sophisticated measures of the incidence and prevalence of disease, including trends over time. GPS and electronic media have added to the timeliness of such measures.

Epidemiology is relevant to hospital engagement with the community because it provides well-established measures to use in planning and evaluating hospital performance (Fleming 2008). The CDC is the nation's leading government public health agency. Directly and indirectly, the CDC has contributed to the emergence of public health as a measurable discipline. This enables hospitals to move community activity from "random acts of kindness" to a highly precise activity with a community impact that can be measured for process performance as well as short-term and long-term outcomes. Logic models (Exhibit 2.2) are widely employed by public health experts to show

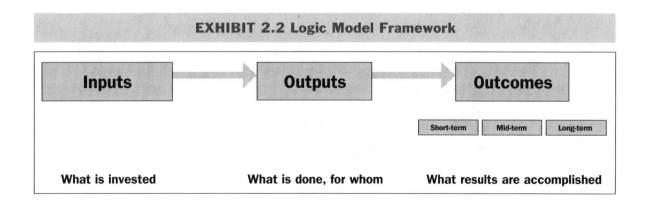

EXHIBIT 2.2 Logic Model Framework

Inputs → Outputs → Outcomes

Short-term   Mid-term   Long-term

What is invested   What is done, for whom   What results are accomplished the relationships between external factors and inputs for achieving short-term and long-term outcomes in ameliorating diseases and chronic conditions (Frechtling 2007). An entire field of public health informatics has emerged (AMIA 2012). As public health has become an evidence-based field, it has enabled other healthcare entities, including hospitals, to take advantage of measurement science to identify, select, and evaluate the activities that are likely to have the greatest impact on the health status of the community (Brownson et al. 2011; IOM 2011).

Epidemiology also enables hospitals to analyze the health problems of their communities in great detail. Describing one's community using disease-specific aggregate data based on time-lagged information reported to the state or decennial census data is no longer acceptable.

Measures of Community Health Status

Sophisticated ways to measure the health status of a community are emerging, which then facilitate measuring the impact of different interventions and comparing their relative effectiveness.

One example of applying public health science to hospital activities is in the area of screenings. The CDC operates the Community Guide (www.thecommunityguide.org), a website that compares the evidence-based effectiveness of a long list of screenings for many specific subpopulations. For hospitals that regularly engage in community health fairs and offer free or reduced-price screenings, this website is invaluable for pinpointing screenings that will be appropriate for the target population and those that will be a waste of time and money. For example, the Community Guide (CDC 2012b) uses the evidence available from high-quality research studies to compare and rate different types of cancer screenings—as they apply to defined subgroups—as "recommended," "recommended against," or "insufficient evidence" (Exhibit 2.3). For those screenings found to be effective, the Community Guide includes evaluations of their economic efficiency (costs).

The CDC has compiled a broader list of frequently recommended health outcomes and determinants (CDC 2013). Starting with a logic model of factors influencing health status, the CDC analyzed ten seminal sources of meta-analyses that analyzed 42 factors (determinants) that either directly affect morbidity and

Interventions for clients either provide education to increase cancer screening or make it easier for clients to be screened. Results are reported separately for breast, cervical, and colorectal cancer screening because routine screening recommendations differ by age and sex.

Task Force Recommendations and Findings

This table lists interventions reviewed by The Community Guide, with Task Force findings for each.

Interventions	Breast Cancer	Cervical Cancer	Colorectal Cancer
Client Reminders	Recommended July 2010	Recommended July 2010	Recommended July 2010
Client Incentives	Insufficient Evidence July 2010	Insufficient Evidence July 2010	Insufficient Evidence July 2010
Small Media	Recommended December 2005	Recommended December 2005	Recommended December 2005
Mass Media	Insufficient Evidence October 2009	Insufficient Evidence October 2009	Insufficient Evidence October 2009
Group Education	Recommended October 2009	Insufficient Evidence October 2009	Insufficient Evidence October 2009
One-on-One Education	Recommended March 2010	Recommended March 2010	Recommended March 2010
Reducing Structural Barriers	Recommended March 2010	Insufficient Evidence March 2010	Recommended March 2010
Reducing Client Out-of-Pocket Costs	Recommended October 2009	Insufficient Evidence October 2009	Insufficient Evidence October 2009

SOURCE: CDC (2012c).

mortality or affect factors known to affect morbidity and mortality. The result is a highly condensed guide to activities targeted at either communities or individuals that will improve overall community health status. Using such data-based studies can help hospitals allocate scarce resources to achieve the greatest effectiveness. A classic example is the emergency department that treats a child successfully for acute asthma attacks but neither asks about nor follows up to address home conditions and behaviors that will prevent future emergencies. The CDC determinants guide is one resource for identifying initiatives in the community that would have a significant return in community health improvement.

The Agency for Healthcare Research and Quality (AHRQ) has supported and examined extensive data on the measurement and effectiveness of various prevention and treatment methods. These data have been compiled into accessible, searchable databases, including the National Quality Measures Clearinghouse (www.qualitymeasures.ahrq .gov) and the National Guideline Clearinghouse (http://guideline .gov) for evidence-based clinical practice guidelines (AHRQ 2012). The Substance Abuse and Mental Health Services Administration (SAMHSA 2012) has cataloged treatments that are effective for those with behavioral problems in the National Registry of Evidence-based Programs and Practices (www .nrepp.samhsa.gov).

Healthy People is another major government initiative, supported by many private healthcare and public health organizations, to determine the status of the nation's health conditions and to set priorities for the future (HHS 2012). Healthy People began in the 1980s with its first national goals set for 2000. The goals—which include 42 major topic areas, 600 objectives, and 1,200 measures—are revised each decade; the 2010 goals are now past, and goals for 2020 are in place. The objectives set target rates of incidence or prevalence, based on current statistics and realistic programs for achieving change. The large list has been narrowed to leading health indicators to create a pared-down set of 26 indicators pertaining to 12 topics. For example, within the major topic of Nutrition and Weight Status, Objective NW5-9 is "Reduce the proportion of adults who are obese" from 34 percent to 30.6 percent, a 10 percent decrease. The Healthy People website (www.healthypeople.gov) includes targets, data sources for each condition, and a link to research studies pertaining to the condition and its remediation. Although most public health professionals are well aware of the Healthy People program and its goals, many of those working in hospitals, physician practices, and other clinically oriented organizations are not familiar with this initiative and how it can be used to guide and measure hospital activities with the community.

The collective activities of the CDC, the National Institutes of Health, the US Department of Health & Human Services, many state governments, and private initiatives have produced numerous sources of free yet detailed and current data that can be used to assess the health of a community (Exhibit 2.4). County Health Rankings (www .countyhealthrankings.org) is one example of a nationwide database that measures and ranks each county in the United States on characteristics that are known to affect health status. The Health Indicators Warehouse (http://healthindicators.gov) compiles many of these data sets and facilitates easy access to data on a given topic. Hospitals can tap into these data sets, add hospital-specific data, and establish realistic and measurable goals for improving community health status while engaging in programs that are consistent with the hospital's mission and resources.

State and local governments and private sources also gather useful

EXHIBIT 2.4 Free National Data Sources That Include Local Data

Census data: http://quickfacts.census.gov

County data: www.countyhealthrankings.org

National Cancer Institute: www.cancer.gov

Health Indicators Warehouse: http://healthindicators.gov

Behavioral Risk Factor Surveillance System: www.cdc.gov/brfss

Mental health and substance abuse: www.nrepp.samhsa.gov

Community Guide: www.thecommunityguide.org

Agency for Healthcare Research and Quality National Quality Measures Clearinghouse: www.qualitymeasures.ahrq.gov

Healthy People: www.healthypeople.gov

data relevant to community health status, much of which is available at no charge. The National Association of County and City Health Officials (NACCHO 2013) engages in a range of programs that often include data collection about community health status as well as workforce and local surveillance trends. The Healthy Communities Institute (2012) in Northern California has created a sophisticated dashboard for tracking changes in community health status based on automatic input of county-level data. This dashboard is used by a consortium of organizations so that the individual and collective contributions to community targets can be measured over time. Dignity Health, in partnership with Truven Health, has created its own data system, the Community Need Index, for measuring community health for its member institutions (Barsi 2009). These measures are incorporated into the strategic plan for each institution, and progress is tracked and reported annually as part of the performance report of individual healthcare executives as well as reported to each community. The top-level data and community mapping are available for free at www.dignityhealth.org/cni.

REALISTIC EXPECTATIONS

One caveat is that changing the health of an entire community requires time. A hospital—and its community partners—must allow time for changes to take place. This process includes educating the public, changing individual and institutional behaviors, implementing monitoring systems, and tracking trends over time. Some changes, such as vaccination rates and the diseases they prevent, can be measured immediately and the impact projected with relative accuracy. Other activities, such as sun protection, are more difficult to measure. Moreover, since skin cancer can take 30 years to develop, outcome measures are less precise or require a realistic expectation of the length of time required for the disease pattern to change.

A second consideration is that the attribution of results to collaborative versus individual efforts is often challenged. Where direct impact cannot clearly be ascribed to the actions of an individual institution, having the hospital select evidence-based activities for which outcomes can be measured is all the more important.

ACTIONS FOR HEALTHCARE EXECUTIVES

- Become familiar with the measures available for monitoring the health status of the community.
- Define the demographic and health status of the community or communities the hospital serves in detail using current data, including a bigger picture than just the patients served by the hospital.
- Apply the principles of evidence-based healthcare management to selecting and prioritizing the hospital's activities with each community it serves.
- Set realistic but measurable goals and objectives for the hospital's community engagement.
- Tap into data sources from public health and other national databases to analyze the health of the hospital's community and to evaluate the hospital's role.

CHAPTER 3

Community Benefit

*C*ommunity benefit (CB), as defined for this book, refers to the Internal Revenue Service (IRS) requirement that nonprofit hospitals must report in detail how they benefit their communities to maintain their tax-exempt status (IRS 2012a). Few senior-level healthcare executives have been immersed in formal CB programming. The regulation instituted by the IRS in 2008 has forced more healthcare executives to become familiar with the reporting requirements, if not the CB activities themselves. Moreover, the concept of the hospital's responsibility for community health was reinforced by additional provisions in the Patient Protection and Affordable Care Act of 2010 (ACA). As regulations go into effect and more details unfold through IRS notices, healthcare executives must understand the provisions of both tax exemption and legal compliance.

A critical component of these changes is that the detailed reports to the IRS are publicly available. In the past, a hospital could engage in whatever community-oriented activities it chose and report in whatever format it wanted to highlight its contributions. The IRS now requires detailed reporting of elements that the hospital might previously not have made public. This new transparency places the hospital, its executives, and its board under scrutiny.

This chapter highlights IRS Form 990 Schedule H requirements. Chapter 4 addresses the obligations of tax-exempt hospitals regarding community health needs assessments (CHNAs) and community health improvement plans (CHIPs) as specified by the ACA. Examining the IRS forms line by line can be tedious, but each line has underlying implications for hospital management. Experienced senior executives will appreciate the complexity of the process and the data required to fill in each line of the form. They can then determine if their organization is acting efficiently and accurately in handling programming as well as completing the form. The issues are relevant to all types

of hospitals, regardless of reporting mandates, as they have changed what communities expect from their hospitals.

An important note: Despite the threat of withholding tax-exempt status, the current IRS regulations specify no dollar amounts or other metrics of performance. (The minor exception is a small fine for not completing the CHNA on time—see Chapter 4 for more detail.) Whether or not a hospital is providing "enough" benefit to its community to warrant tax exemption is not currently evaluated. This puts the burden of commitment on hospital executive leadership and governance.

HISTORY OF COMMUNITY BENEFIT

Hospitals have always been integral parts of their communities, as noted in Chapter 1. How they contribute to their communities became a separate issue when tax exemption was awarded. As the federal tax code developed in the 1950s and 1960s, hospitals were granted exemption from federal taxes on the premise that they offer benefits to their communities in lieu of paying taxes and on the assumption that if the hospital did not provide certain services, the government would need to do so. (This philosophy was also evident as the underpinning of the Hill-Burton Act.) The language was general, and no criteria were specified for measuring the benefit or the penalties for failing to comply. Most states automatically extended the tax exemption to state taxes as well.

The history of compliance with tax-exemption requirements has been documented in detail elsewhere (CBO 2006). The IRS provided a revenue ruling in 1969 (69-545) that stated the basis for hospital tax exemption as "contribution to the community." For most hospitals, charity care was the primary source of community benefit. The American Hospital Association developed The Community Benefit Standard in the late 1980s, describing the "gold standard" of CB (Seay and Sigmond 1989)—but this was never formally adopted or recognized by the IRS. As occasional challenges to hospitals' tax exemption arose, the Catholic Health Association (CHA) initiated its Social Accountability Budget to delineate and report the myriad ways that nonprofit healthcare organizations contribute to their communities beyond charity care (CHA 1989). Meanwhile, over the years, 18 states implemented various laws or regula-

tions to ensure that nonprofit hospitals were indeed earning the right to tax exemption through the variety of ways they contributed to their community's health (Community Catalyst 2007).

Lack of definition, variation in activities, lack of nationwide data, and above all, lack of societal interest allowed hospitals to define their own portfolio of community activities. Charity care was the dominant type of CB. Health education, screenings, and health promotion projects were also typical. Few hospitals had formal CB departments, and the activities considered outreach to the community were often organized by the marketing, public relations, mission, or health education departments.

In the 1990s and early 2000s, Senator Charles Grassley (R-Iowa) and others repeatedly challenged the validity of hospitals' claims to tax exemption (Senate Committee on Finance 2007). The Government Accountability Office (GAO 2008), Congressional Budget Office (CBO 2006), and IRS (2007) produced reports, and the Senate held hearings to examine hospitals' activities with regard to the community. The result for nonprofit hospitals was the addition of Schedule H to IRS Form 990, which nonprofit organizations are required to submit to the IRS as part of their annual tax return.

SCHEDULE H IMPLEMENTATION

Schedule H is a six-part form on which nonprofit hospitals report the ways in which they contribute to their communities (see Exhibit 3.1). Several types of financial assistance combined as "charity care" make up the single largest component and represent the vast majority of dollars reported—although the exact percentage and dollar amounts remain to be determined once data from Schedule H become widely available.

Preliminary reporting of Schedule H began in 2008 as optional. Full reporting was deferred from 2009 until 2010. Depending on the hospital's fiscal year, complete reporting for many hospitals did not occur until calendar year 2011. Meanwhile, the IRS monitored the early experience and sought comments on various components of the form. The ACA, passed in 2010, directly affected both CB activities and their reporting. Schedule H was further revised in 2011, with much more detail added on financial assistance and CHNAs.

The full version of Schedule H and current reporting instructions are available online (www.irs.gov/pub/irs-pdf/f990sh.pdf) with 18 detailed pages of instructions (www.irs.gov/pub/irs-pdf/i990sh.pdf). A summary of the main elements is presented in this chapter so that senior executives can appreciate the magnitude of the operational changes inherent in completing the new Schedule H and managing a comprehensive CB program. The practical implications of Schedule H are that hospitals can no longer consider CB as a perfunctory function fulfilled primarily by uncompensated care. The nature of the activities has changed from "random acts of kindness" to deliberate efforts to apply an evidence-based approach to activities conducted outside the walls of the hospital. Moreover, the complexity of the reporting requires participation and collaboration by numerous hospital departments and individuals.

SIX COMPONENTS OF SCHEDULE H

Schedule H contains six different parts, described here with sufficient detail to show the breadth of impact on management functions. The form has already evolved, as both

EXHIBIT 3.1 Schedule H, Form 990 Overview

Part I: Community Benefit–Financial Assistance

    Lines 1–5: Financial Assistance Policies

    Line 6: Community Benefit (CB) Reporting

    Line 7: Financial Assistance

        a. At cost

        b. Medicaid

        c. Cost of other means-tested government programs

        d. Total financial assistance (7a–7c)

        e. Community health improvement and CB operations

        f. Health professions education

        g. Subsidized health services

        h. Research

        i. Cash and in-kind contributions

        j. Total (7e–7i)

        k. Total (7d and 7j)

Part II: Community-Building Activities

Part III: Bad Debt, Medicare, and Collection Practices

Part IV: Management Companies and Joint Ventures

Part V: Facility Information

Part VI: Supplemental Information

SOURCE: IRS (2012a).

hospitals and the IRS gain a better understanding of what information is meaningful and how to gather it.

Part I: Financial Assistance and Certain Other Community Benefits

Financial assistance to those uninsured, underinsured, or unable to pay for their medical care has long been viewed as the most important way that a hospital contributes to the well-being of its community. For many years, this category was referred to in the aggregate as *charity care*. The passage of the ACA has increased attention on financial access to healthcare. Much more emphasis is now placed on the broader category of *financial assistance* and the hospital's relevant policies.

Part I of Schedule H, lines 1 through 6 (Exhibit 3.2), as well as some subsequent sections, requires that hospitals report about their financial assistance policies, what criteria they contain, and how they are applied and publicized. But checking the simple *yes* or *no* questions involves much more complicated analysis and accountability for the CEO and hospital board. For example, question 4 asks, "Did the organization's financial assistance policy that applied to the largest number of its patients during the tax year provide for free or discounted care to the 'medically indigent'?" Question 5c asks, "As a result of budget considerations, was the organization unable to provide free or discounted care to a patient who was eligible for free or discounted care?" These one-liners exceed what the typical hospital financial report contains. They require knowledge about the intersection of the hospital's financial policy and its criteria for assistance, the hospital budget, data gathered about individual patients, and payment sources for individuals falling into specific categories. Moreover, if the hospital checks *yes*, then it is subject to members of the community and other stakeholders asking tough questions, such as Who was denied free or discounted care? Why? Why was the budget inadequate?

How financial policies are communicated to patients and the community, as well as how they are implemented, receives increased attention on Schedule H. A policy written in English posted on a door or website is not likely to be seen or understood by some of the people most likely to need financial assistance. Ongoing training of the financial assistance staff members is essential so that they stay informed of changes

EXHIBIT 3.2 Schedule H, Part I

SCHEDULE H (Form 990)	Hospitals	OMB No. 1545-0047
	▶ Complete if the organization answered "Yes" to Form 990, Part IV, question 20. ▶ Attach to Form 990. ▶ See separate instructions.	2011
Department of the Treasury Internal Revenue Service		Open to Public Inspection

Name of the organization		Employer identification number

Part I   Financial Assistance and Certain Other Community Benefits at Cost

			Yes	No
1a	Did the organization have a financial assistance policy during the tax year? If "No," skip to question 6a . .	**1a**		
b	If "Yes," was it a written policy?	**1b**		
2	If the organization had multiple hospital facilities, indicate which of the following best describes application of the financial assistance policy to its various hospital facilities during the tax year.			
	☐ Applied uniformly to all hospital facilities ☐ Applied uniformly to most hospital facilities ☐ Generally tailored to individual hospital facilities			
3	Answer the following based on the financial assistance eligibility criteria that applied to the largest number of the organization's patients during the tax year.			
a	Did the organization use Federal Poverty Guidelines (FPG) to determine eligibility for providing *free* care? If "Yes," indicate which of the following was the FPG family income limit for eligibility for free care:	**3a**		
	☐ 100% ☐ 150% ☐ 200% ☐ Other _____ %			
b	Did the organization use FPG to determine eligibility for providing *discounted* care? If "Yes," indicate which of the following was the family income limit for eligibility for discounted care:	**3b**		
	☐ 200% ☐ 250% ☐ 300% ☐ 350% ☐ 400% ☐ Other _____ %			
c	If the organization did not use FPG to determine eligibility, describe in Part VI the income based criteria for determining eligibility for free or discounted care. Include in the description whether the organization used an asset test or other threshold, regardless of income, to determine eligibility for free or discounted care.			
4	Did the organization's financial assistance policy that applied to the largest number of its patients during the tax year provide for free or discounted care to the "medically indigent"?	**4**		
5a	Did the organization budget amounts for free or discounted care provided under its financial assistance policy during the tax year?	**5a**		
b	If "Yes," did the organization's financial assistance expenses exceed the budgeted amount?	**5b**		
c	If "Yes" to line 5b, as a result of budget considerations, was the organization unable to provide free or discounted care to a patient who was eligible for free or discounted care?	**5c**		
6a	Did the organization prepare a community benefit report during the tax year?	**6a**		
b	If "Yes," did the organization make it available to the public?	**6b**		
	Complete the following table using the worksheets provided in the Schedule H instructions. Do not submit these worksheets with the Schedule H.			

SOURCE: IRS (2012a).

and fine points of application. Language barriers require extra efforts to address, especially if a patient signed forms upon admission without fully understanding the payment process or his obligations.

Lines 7a through 7d (Exhibit 3.3) require the hospital to report on other means-tested government programs for the number of people served, total expense, direct offsetting revenue, net expense, and per-

EXHIBIT 3.3 Schedule H: Reporting of Activities and Programs

7	Financial Assistance and Certain Other Community Benefits at Cost						
	Financial Assistance and Means-Tested Government Programs	**(a)** Number of activities or programs (optional)	**(b)** Persons served (optional)	**(c)** Total community benefit expense	**(d)** Direct offsetting revenue	**(e)** Net community benefit expense	**(f)** Percent of total expense
a	Financial Assistance at cost (from Worksheet 1) . . .						
b	Medicaid (from Worksheet 3, column a)						
c	Costs of other means-tested government programs (from Worksheet 3, column b)						
d	**Total** Financial Assistance and Means-Tested Government Programs						
	Other Benefits						
e	Community health improvement services and community benefit operations (from Worksheet 4) .						
f	Health professions education (from Worksheet 5)						
g	Subsidized health services (from Worksheet 6)						
h	Research (from Worksheet 7) .						
i	Cash and in-kind contributions for community benefit (from Worksheet 8)						
j	**Total.** Other Benefits						
k	**Total.** Add lines 7d and 7j . .						

For Paperwork Reduction Act Notice, see the Instructions for Form 990. Cat. No. 50192T Schedule H (Form 990) 2011

SOURCE: IRS (2012a).

cent of the hospital's total expense. These numbers are more likely to be readily available as part of the hospital's existing financial statements, but they must be compiled on Schedule H to be consistent with what is reported elsewhere and with each other. The IRS provides worksheets to facilitate completion.

Lines 7e through 7i (Exhibit 3.3) are other one-liners that require input far more extensive than is apparent. The categories themselves

are broad: community health improvement services, community benefit operations, health professions education, subsidized health services, research, cash, and in-kind community benefit. For each category, the hospital must report the number of activities or programs, the total expense, any direct offsetting revenue, the net expense, and the percent of total expense; reporting the number of persons served is optional. Although the IRS Form

990 Schedule H Instructions provide worksheets, the amount of information to be gathered and reported in a systematic way can be immense.

For example, just reporting on health professions education potentially requires compiling information from multiple departments, including nursing, allied health, graduate medical education (GME), medical education, and continuing education. Expenses for each category must be apportioned between activities that count as community benefit and those that do not count. If the nursing education unit offers only continuing education courses that are open to all nurses in the community, then the salaries of the staff working on these programs can be taken in totality as valid expenses. If, however, the nursing education unit offers some classes only for nurses employed by the hospital, then these do not count as CB because they benefit only the single institution and not the broader community. In calculating the expenses reported, the salary of each person then needs to be allocated by some acceptable formula to those classes that do count and exclude staff time spent on classes that do not count. In short, the total unit budget cannot be directly applied to CB because only some of the activities are deemed

acceptable under IRS guidance. Offsetting revenues must be deducted, including the amount the hospital receives from Medicare and Medicaid for direct GME payments, tuition, and other sundry sources of compensation for education.

Community health improvement services and subsidized health services are two other challenging categories. *Community health improvement services* are defined by the IRS (2012b) as "activities or programs, subsidized by the health care organization, carried out or supported for the express purpose of improving community health. Such services do not generate inpatient or outpatient bills.... Community need for the activity or program must be established." *Subsidized health services* are defined as "clinical services provided despite a financial loss to the organization." Subsidized services are those that are essential to the community and would not be available if not provided by the hospital, the government, or another tax-exempt entity. The hospital might lose money on these services—such as burn units, neonatal intensive care units, and emergency departments—but it provides them because they are essential to the community. The hospital is then allowed to claim losses after various adjustments. However, while the need for some services is obvious, others, such as skilled nursing or home health, might be challenged. If the hospital did not offer skilled nursing, would a proprietary chain enter to fill this void?

Research can be itemized as a CB, provided it is funded by a tax-exempt or government entity or funded by the hospital itself, and the results are made publicly available. Research conducted for internal purposes only, such as quality improvement, is not considered CB.

Cash donations and in-kind contributions are recognized as CB but cannot include capital. A hospital that routinely donates its used imaging equipment to a community health center would not be able to take credit for this donation, even if the community health center depends on the imaging equipment to offer vital services. (This example should be kept in mind when considering what and how the hospital reports its CB to the community.) The hospital can continue to donate its used equipment, but the value of the donation cannot be considered as an in-kind CB contribution. These donations can be reported in Section VI as "other" contributions.

In the past, the financial statements made public by hospitals did not necessarily reveal in such detail how expenses were allocated or revenues accrued. The new reporting forces hospitals to identify services that lose money, at least in aggregate, and services offered as efforts to improve community health. This reporting subjects the hospital to challenges from the IRS, other providers, or the community about the appropriateness of its financial and programmatic decisions. This visibility is one of the major reasons the executive leadership and board must be aware of what is reported on Form 990 and the underlying composition of the service profile and accounting methodology.

Part II: Community Building

The original version of Schedule H required the reporting of community building activities, but they did not count toward fulfilling community obligations (CHA 2008). In the 2011 revision, the IRS acknowledged that community-building activities do indeed contribute to the community's health and well-being and therefore should count, but they are reported separately (Exhibit 3.4). (Recall that at least at the present, no dollar amounts or percentages have been

EXHIBIT 3.4 Schedule H: Reporting Community-Building Activities

Part II **Community Building Activities** Complete this table if the organization conducted any community building activities during the tax year, and describe in Part VI how its community building activities promoted the health of the communities it serves.

		(a) Number of activities or programs (optional)	(b) Persons served (optional)	(c) Total community building expense	(d) Direct offsetting revenue	(e) Net community building expense	(f) Percent of total expense
1	Physical improvements and housing						
2	Economic development						
3	Community support						
4	Environmental improvements						
5	Leadership development and training for community members						
6	Coalition building						
7	Community health improvement advocacy						
8	Workforce development						
9	Other						
10	**Total**						

SOURCE: IRS (2012a).

set as a requirement for tax exemption, so the issue of counting versus not counting is moot. However, these requirements may be forthcoming.)

Community-building activities include outreach efforts related to

- Physical improvements and housing
- Economic development
- Community support
- Environmental improvements
- Leadership development and training for community members
- Coalition building
- Community health improvement advocacy
- Workforce development
- Other programs

This obviously broad list allows the hospital to include the expenses of activities ranging from lead abatement programs to hosting meetings of community health coalitions to subsidizing day care centers. The IRS instructions provide examples of activities for each category, but these are not exhaustive and allow the hospital to define what constitutes community building for its unique situation.

In Part VI, the hospital must justify how the activities reported in

Part II benefit the community. This is where the intersection of program activities and measurements of their impact becomes imperative. The CDC determinants guide discussed in Chapter 2 offers one potential source of justification for some community-building activities. Lead abatement projects, for example, relate to housing, a subject included in the CDC analysis under "physical environment" determinants of health. The hospital's justification for the lead abatement project would then include a reference to CDC research.

Completing Part II requires combing the hospital for myriad seemingly unrelated activities, calculating detailed expenses, and then combining the data in a way that rolls up to a single line for each category, and ultimately, to the totals of line 10. Exhibit 3.5 gives an example of the information that would be needed to report accurately on a single meeting hosted by the hospital for a community coalition.

Community building requires deliberation and selection. On one hand, a community hospital might have dozens of activities throughout the year that could be counted. On the other hand, each activity must then be justified with a statement, and preferably metrics, about how it contributes to the community. Moreover, the staff time required to calculate the attendance, expenses, and revenue elements might arguably exceed the value of reporting. Hospitals that provide large dollar amounts of financial assistance reported in Part I could well decide not to report anything under Part II, which would reduce the time and effort required to complete Schedule H as well as the risk of data errors. The downside of opting not to report anything in Part II is the transparency of the report to the community.

Part III: Bad Debt, Medicare, and Collection Practices

Part III asks for more information about how the hospital manages financial affairs, including bad debt, Medicare, and debt collection.

Under Section A, the hospital must report bad debt and Medicare shortfalls. The IRS assumes use of Healthcare Financial Management Association (HFMA) Statement No. 15 as guidance for reporting bad debt (HFMA 2006). Hospitals that do *not* use HFMA Statement No. 15 must explain what they use instead. Moreover, a hospital must report the amount of bad debt, the footnote of the hospital's financial statement

EXHIBIT 3.5 Reporting a Community-Building Activity

A hospital can count meetings hosted on behalf of the community toward its CB as community support, coalition building, or community health improvement advocacy—depending on the purpose of the meeting. To report costs completely and accurately, the hospital must record the following information:

- Purpose of the meeting
- Number of people attending the meeting from the community
- Number of people attending the meeting from the hospital
- For each hospital staff member who attended, length of participation (hours) and salary, to calculate value of total staff attendance
- Staff time devoted to marketing, planning, and coordinating logistics, by hours of contribution, by hourly salary of staff involved
- Size of room (square feet)
- Maintenance cost per square foot for the relevant building, to calculate value of room
- AV equipment used
- Value of AV equipment used and length of time in use
- Support services rendered (e.g., special security for a night meeting)
- Food and beverages provided
- Food-per-person cost multiplied by number of people attending
- Number of parking vouchers given and cost per voucher
- Photocopying, number of pages multiplied by cost per page
- Any other direct expenses covered by the hospital or indirect expenses

For each such meeting the hospital hosts, similar details must be recorded. These are then aggregated into a single line on IRS Form 990 Schedule H, Part II, line 3 or line 6.

that describes bad debt, the costing methodology used, the relationship of bad debt to financial assistance policy application, and the rationale for why bad debt should be considered a CB.

Section B pertains specifically to Medicare. Again, the hospital must report revenue, allowable costs, surplus or shortfall, costing methodology, and the rationale for considering any shortfall to be CB.

Section C asks about collection policies, including the relationship of collection policy to financial assistance policies.

Although Part III asks for only five numbers and three *yes* or *no* answers, its contents indicate how complex Schedule H reporting has become. Cost reporting methods and financial policies must be incorporated into the seemingly simple answers. Data and accounting methodologies used to report CB should be consistent with those the hospital uses to report to Medicare and Medicaid—although Schedule H instructions provide worksheets that allow the hospital to calculate a cost–charges ratio that can be used for reporting specifically on Schedule H. And, although the hospital's finance department can be assumed to have the numbers to complete this section, the units that deal with application of policies might include third-party collection agencies that must now be counted on to apply the hospital's collection policy to reflect its financial assistance policies as well.

Part IV: Management Companies and Joint Ventures

Part IV offers a bit of a break—provided a hospital understands the definitions inherent in the question. (The IRS provides a glossary of definitions for Schedule H as well as instructions.) This section asks the hospital to report management companies and joint ventures, including percentage of ownership for the organization, the directors, trustees, key employees, and physicians. The intent of this section is to ensure that the hospital has fulfilled the spirit of a nonprofit entity rather than sheltering financial benefits by creating diversified organizational structures.

Part V: Facility Information

Part V asks about the entities that are part of the hospital's legal organization. The reporting entity is whatever legal organization holds the tax ID number. For the most part, the IRS deems individual hospitals to be responsible for meeting their obligation to their community. This prevents health systems from pooling their resources or reporting on the hospitals' activities or their communities' needs on an aggregate basis.

The first (2008) version of Part V was just a list of key hospital services and number of beds. The 2011 version has expanded Part V to three and a half pages of detail that repeat some of the information asked in previous sections. For each entity that is reported under the hospital's tax ID number, the hospital must report in Section A the existence of several services and the number of medical and surgical beds. Section B now requires detailed information for each entity about CHNAs (covered in Chapter 4), financial assistance policies, billing and collection policies, and emergency department policies.

Part VI: Supplemental Information

Part VI of Schedule H, along with Section B in Part V, overlaps with the ACA. The 2011 revision adds extensive detail to the 2008 version of Part VI, which was primarily an open-ended place for the hospital to report information it believed to be essential to justify its contributions to the community. Part VI (Exhibit 3.6) is brief—only seven questions—but it requires justification and explanation of everything that has come before it—and then some. Line 1, for example, requests: "Provide the descriptions required for Part I, lines 3c, 6a,

---

EXHIBIT 3.6 Schedule H: Reporting Supplemental Activity

Schedule H (Form 990) 2011   Page **8**

Part VI Supplemental Information

Complete this part to provide the following information.

1   **Required descriptions.** Provide the descriptions required for Part I, lines 3c, 6a, and 7; Part II; Part III, lines 4, 8, and 9b; and Part V, Section B, lines 1j, 3, 4, 5c, 6i, 7, 9, 10, 11h, 13g, 15e, 16e, 17e, 18d, 19d, 20, and 21.

2   **Needs assessment.** Describe how the organization assesses the health care needs of the communities it serves, in addition to any needs assessments reported in Part V, Section B.

3   **Patient education of eligibility for assistance.** Describe how the organization informs and educates patients and persons who may be billed for patient care about their eligibility for assistance under federal, state, or local government programs or under the organization's financial assistance policy.

4   **Community information.** Describe the community the organization serves, taking into account the geographic area and demographic constituents it serves.

5   **Promotion of community health.** Provide any other information important to describing how the organization's hospital facilities or other health care facilities further its exempt purpose by promoting the health of the community (e.g., open medical staff, community board, use of surplus funds, etc.).

6   **Affiliated health care system.** If the organization is part of an affiliated health care system, describe the respective roles of the organization and its affiliates in promoting the health of the communities served.

7   **State filing of community benefit report.** If applicable, identify all states with which the organization, or a related organization, files a community benefit report.

SOURCE: IRS (2012a).

and 7; Part II; Part III, lines 4, 8, and 9b; and Part V, Section B, lines 1j, 3, 4, 5c, 6i, 7, 9, 10, 11h, 13g, 15e, 16e, 17e, 18d, 19d, 20, and 2l." Several of the items relate to CHNAs; these are discussed in Chapter 4.

Line 5 reads, "Provide any other information important to describing how the organization's hospital facilities or other health care facilities further its exempt purpose by promoting the health of the community." Although the form gives examples such as "open medical staff, community board, use of surplus funds," the hospital can use metrics here to measure and report its success in improving community health. For example, as mentioned in Chapter 2, Part VI enables the hospital to demonstrate the value of using an evidence-based approach to selecting and evaluating which activities compose its CB program. This question also offers the hospital the opportunity to report on programs or services to communities other than those the hospital has defined for IRS reporting purposes. For example, contributions of supplies or clinical expertise or equipment to developing countries that are consistent with the hospital's mission can be reported here, regardless of the IRS not count-

ing these activities when considering the hospital's tax exemption.

COMPLETING SCHEDULE H

The mechanics of completing Schedule H have serious implications for hospital operations. Before Schedule H, a hospital needed no formal report. Catholic entities might have chosen to use the Community Benefit Inventory for Social Accountability (CBISA) to track their activities, but with no financial or legal repercussions, the social accountability form could be filled out by one person, who might be a staff member in the mission, community health, or marketing department. The amount of information, detail, and precision reported on Schedule H now requires active involvement from staff responsible for biomedical research, patient education, continuing education, finance, residency training, accounting, nursing services, building maintenance, and other departments. The accounting department staff members are not likely to know enough programmatic information to complete the form unilaterally; conversely, the program staff are not likely to be sufficiently familiar with accounting and financial policies to complete the form. Because reporting CB now is a legal requirement, ballpark estimates or blanks are not acceptable, and the hospital does not want to exclude activities because of a lack of data. Moreover, if each department or unit involved provides its own response, the hospital's overall report might lack cohesion, consistency, and comprehensiveness.

In short, completing Schedule H requires the hospital to reconcile the goal of efficient delegation of duties with the old saying that "a camel is a giraffe drawn by a committee." One aid is the emergence of accounting systems designed specifically to report CB, including compliance with IRS regulations, definitions, and format, that can accommodate input from staff from any unit in the hospital.

ACTIONS FOR HEALTHCARE EXECUTIVES

- Review financial assistance policies for content, communication, and staff knowledge; ensure that they are being followed.
- Review and monitor bad debt and collection policies and practices

for content, communication, and implementation, particularly if the collections function is outsourced.
- Monitor Schedule H completion—who is filling it out and how, and what checks and balances are in place to ensure accuracy, completeness, and consistency.
- Examine internal coordination of all departments and units contributing to CB activities so that the full magnitude of the hospital's efforts can be realized.
- Make sure that someone in the line of CB accountability and authority is monitoring ongoing modifications to Schedule H, for example through membership in the Association for Community Health Improvement, Catholic Health Association, or a similar advocacy group that regularly updates members about CB regulations.
- Share the annual CB plan and report with the hospital board.
- Gather information such that the legally reported document can be translated into a report that is compelling to lay consumers and other stakeholders.

CHAPTER 4

Community Health Needs Assessments and Implementation Plans

The Patient Protection and Affordable Care Act (ACA 2010, 125 Stat 119) mandates that hospitals wishing to retain tax-exempt status engage in three spheres of activities: financial assistance policies and practices; emergency care, billing, and collection policies and practices; and community health needs assessments (CHNAs) and the resulting community health implementation plan (CHIP). These activities relate to community benefit programming as described in Chapter 3 but are distinct in that they are incorporated into the law rather than articulated only in regulations. Charge notification practices and collection policies are discussed in Chapter 3. This chapter covers the essential elements of CHNAs and CHIPs.

COMMUNITY HEALTH NEEDS ASSESSMENTS AND IMPLEMENTATION PLANS

Section 9007(a) of the ACA added sections 501(r) and 4959 to the federal tax code and amended section 6033(b)—all of which specify requirements for hospitals. The new law mandates that hospitals with 501(c)(3) tax-exempt status comply with several provisions related to the health needs of the community. The hospital must conduct a CHNA at least once every three years. The first CHNA will be due in the tax year that follows March 23, 2012—which means that most hospitals will need to have completed it by calendar year 2014. An assessment conducted in the previous two years would also be acceptable. A hospital may use a needs assessment widely accepted by the community, conduct its own needs assessment, conduct a needs assessment in conjunction with other organizations serving the community, or use a combination of methods. In conducting the CHNA, the hospital must:

- involve people with "special knowledge of or expertise in public health,"
- involve persons who represent the broad interests of the community served by the hospital, and
- make the CHNA available to the public, primarily through web posting.

The CHNA must then be used to formulate a CHIP that

- addresses priority needs or explains why priority needs are not being met, and
- is accepted by the governing board by the end of the same tax year as the tax year in which the CHNA was conducted.

The hospital must submit the CHNA and CHIP to the Internal Revenue Service (IRS) with the annual Form 990. The CHNA and CHIP are good for three years, and the same documents may be submitted for each of these years. However, if the hospital fails to complete and submit the CHNA and CHIP, Section 4959 of the tax code (added by the ACA) imposes a $50,000 excise tax on the hospital for each year of noncompliance. State laws must also be considered, as they might have different requirements.

These requirements apply to any hospital that seeks tax exemption under Section 501(c)(3). Government hospitals are excluded from the reporting requirements, but, if they maintain 501(c)(3) entities in addition to the hospital itself—for example, for purposes related to but other than acute inpatient care—they may be required to comply. Health systems owning or operating several hospitals are required to have a distinct CHNA and CHIP for each hospital. The only exception, as of mid-2012, is that multiple hospitals operated with the same federal tax ID number are allowed to file a single report under that ID. For-profit hospitals obviously need not comply. However, with the attention that CHNAs are being given by communities, for-profit hospitals might choose to conduct a CHNA to maintain goodwill, have access to current information, and ensure market acceptance.

Nonprofit hospitals report 501(r) compliance with the CHNA and CHIP using the annual Form 990, Schedule H. At present, the IRS asks about process but specifies neither a set process nor format or content of the intended implementation plan. Details of how hospitals must comply and what they must report continue to evolve.

COMMUNITY HEALTH NEEDS ASSESSMENTS

CHNAs are not new to communities or hospitals. Hospitals have been working with their communities for years to understand needs and meet them within the context of available resources. Catholic healthcare, for example, is replete with examples of religious sisters working in communities to promote well-being, identifying myriad health needs, and establishing hospitals to meet those needs. Kaiser Permanente grew out of Kaiser Industries' recognition of the need for employees to have access to physician care, hospitals, and health insurance.

Previous federal initiatives have required hospitals to assess the needs of their communities. For example, the Comprehensive Health Planning Law of 1966 required hospitals to document the need in the community prior to authorizing new equipment or new services.

For years, states such as California have had community benefit laws that require the hospital to conduct CHNAs. In one model that evolved in California, all of the hospitals in a community work together to conduct a single needs assessment instead of several such needs assessments (see

EXHIBIT 4.1 Examples of Collaborative CHNAs

The State of California implemented SB697 in 1994, requiring that hospitals conduct community health needs assessments and identify top priorities for action. Despite the highly competitive hospital environment of the time, visionary leaders immediately saw the value of hospitals serving a single community working together to maximize use of resources and, more important, to produce a single plan that would lead to a unified approach to ameliorating the most severe community health problems.

In Long Beach, a city of nearly half a million residents, the director of the Long Beach Department of Health and Human Services brought the leaders of the city's major hospitals together and persuaded them to work with the health department to contract with the University of Southern California (USC) for the first major citywide health needs assessment. The (then) Long Beach Memorial Medical Center, Long Beach Community Hospital, and St. Mary Medical Center contributed the financial resources and worked with the health department to engage USC to conduct a CHNA, followed by another three years later. For the third CHNA, the for-profit Pacific Hospital also participated, and the contract to conduct the CHNA was given to the health administration faculty at the local university, California State University, Long Beach (CSULB). Although all the individuals involved in the launch of the collaborative CHNA have changed, this pattern has continued. The Long Beach collaborative has recently completed the sixth citywide CHNA, conducted by the health administration faculty at CSULB.

Exhibit 4.1). The California Health Interview Survey, which began in 2002, grew out of the recognition that all healthcare providers should be working with common data and a shared framework for identifying needs, particularly in areas where myriad small subpopulations make it difficult to ascertain demographic and health condition data from a large enough pool of respondents to achieve statistical significance.

Other nonprofit organizations and government units also conduct CHNAs. The United Way has been the primary leader in many communities. Local health departments must have needs assessments on record in order to apply for accreditation from the Public Health Accreditation Board. Area Agencies on Aging and some government-funded mental health agencies are also mandated to conduct CHNAs.

EXHIBIT 4.2 CHNA Elements Required by the ACA

- Conduct once every three years, with first report due by the end of the first taxable year beginning after March 23, 2012.
- Include input from representatives of the broad community.
- Include input from public health experts.
- Make widely available to the public, including posting on a website.
- Result in a written implementation strategy to address identified needs, with explanation if those needs are not addressed.
- Describe the process used for the CHNA on IRS Form 990, Schedule H, Part VI.
- Pay an excise tax penalty of $50,000 per year for failure to comply.

SOURCE: IRS (2011).

In summary, there is no shortage of CHNAs. However, no single template has emerged. As highlighted in Exhibit 4.2, the IRS has specified some elements that must be incorporated into the conduct of the CHNA. Details for reporting these mandated elements are included in the instructions for reporting Form 990 Schedule H as well as described in IRS Notice 2011-52 (IRS 2011).

With the advent of the ACA requirement has come a flurry of activity by associations and consultants to define how to conduct a valid needs assessment of the community and how to partner with healthcare organizations. Hospital executives should be aware of tools—several of which are listed in the following section—to ensure that CHNAs are methodologically valid, are done efficiently, and involve public health experts and community representatives in such a way that the hospital is beyond criticism. Conversely, hospitals should not be drawn into expensive or overly ambitious efforts. The reporting on Form 990 Schedule H requires only that the hospital describe what it did and how—albeit in some detail.

MODEL HEALTH NEEDS ASSESSMENTS

A CHNA need not be a single study. The CHNA can combine primary data gathered through focus groups, surveys, and key stakeholder interviews. It can use secondary data accessed from existing databases, from hospital patient utilization data to the US Census. The hospital can adopt needs assessments done by other organizations, such as the United Way or the local health department, in total or in part. Managed care and insurance companies may have relevant data. The state health department is a repository for conditions required by law to be reported. Census data and the Centers for Disease Control and Prevention (CDC) now have detailed data available for many communities on demographics, socioeconomic factors that affect health, and health conditions, as described in Chapter 2. The hospital's own data on utilization should also be included.

One of the hospital's challenges is to determine what is available and relevant, and what allocation of resources is necessary to produce a CHNA that is comprehensive and applicable to the hospital.

Resources to guide CHNAs have proliferated since the passage of the ACA. Guides, webinars, conferences, and consultants are readily available. The following are widely known and tend to be well-respected in the field.

MAPP: Mobilizing for Action Through Planning and Partnership. This communitywide strategic planning process is designed to improve community health and strengthen the local public health system, broadly defined to include government public health, community organizations, hospitals, and other healthcare organizations. MAPP has been supported through CDC funding and is driven by the National Association of County and City Health Officials (NACCHO 2012). More information can be found at www.naccho.org.

Community Health Assessment Toolkit. Compiled by the Association for Community Health Improvement (ACHI 2007), this resource is available to members of ACHI, the American Hospital Association (AHA), and the Society for Healthcare Strategy and Market Development at www.assesstoolkit.org.

Assessing and Addressing Community Health Needs. This guidebook was compiled by the Catholic Health Association (CHA) in cooperation with VHA, Inc. and the Healthy Communities Institute (CHA 2011). It details the CHNA process step-by-step and reflects the ACA and IRS regulations.

TIPS FOR CONDUCTING A CHNA

Tips for conducting a CHNA that will meet ACA and IRS regulations include the following:

- Assign explicit responsibility for the CHNA to a single unit within the hospital.
- Find out what exists already and examine it for validity and acceptability to avoid duplicating efforts.
- Identify appropriate partners, including one or more organizations that are widely accepted as representing the community. Include the local health department, as this will also meet the criterion of including persons with expertise in public health.
- Build appropriate infrastructure for incorporating the CHNA into hospital operations. This step is the primary contribution of executive management. The CHNA needs adequate resources, a time frame, an expected product, a report to the hospital board, and a clear impact on the subsequent activities of the hospital.

COMMUNITY HEALTH IMPLEMENTATION PLANS

CHIPs are required of a hospital pursuant to completion of a CHNA. The CHIP must explain what activities the hospital intends to undertake to address the health needs identified through the CHNA. The hospital prioritizes the needs, on the basis of whatever process and criteria it decides, but involving the community is prudent. The hospital must explain on Schedule H, Part VI, how it will address the community health needs deemed to be priorities. For any priority health needs that it will not address, the hospital must explain why. The IRS has provided neither a template for a CHIP nor detailed criteria for the contents or process of prioritizing needs. As of this writing, no CHIPs have yet been submitted, so no tested examples exist. Each hospital thus has the opportunity to determine for itself the content, format, and level of detail it will include in its CHIP. One controversy is whether or not the CHIP must be made public. Hospitals are resisting this step, preferring to gain more experience before publicizing the CHIP. The most recent updates on regulations can be found on the IRS website at www.irs.gov/form990 or from sources such as the AHA or CHA.

CAVEATS

In efforts to comply with new regulations, hospitals should keep in mind that community engagement, community benefit, and CHNAs are intertwined but can also be distinct management initiatives. Who "the community" is and how "community" is defined can vary for different projects. Similarly, the characteristics used for baseline data can be modified to fit the service issues at hand. A given geographic area might have several relevant CHNAs that cover part but not all of the area and some but not all of the target populations. The federal regulations do not insist that the hospital identify only one community, or that funds be spent on community health projects that cover only a single population.

Hospital executives and board members must understand that this flexibility in definition can be both an advantage and a disadvantage. Senior leaders and board members must be able to explain the criteria they use in dealing with community issues, including which CHNAs are endorsed for submission to the IRS and how resources are allocated to address identified needs.

Senior executives also must remember that, whatever guidance the CHNA and CHIP offer about serving the community, executives still have an obligation to exert leadership. A physician who needs new equipment, a staff member who has discovered a new need for a specific service, a community member who appeals for a matching contribu-

tion—all these may be good cases that senior leaders might choose to support regardless of numeric data or formal plans. Transparency and communication, especially between senior staff executives and the board, can help gain support for such decisions. Ultimately, senior executives must assume responsibility for caring for the community and for using the best judgment to steward the community's resources.

ACTIONS FOR HEALTHCARE EXECUTIVES

- Find out the due date for your hospital's CHNA.
- Assign responsibility for the CHNA to a single department, but ensure that other departments that could contribute or benefit from the CHNA are appropriately involved.
- Ask if existing needs assessments have been evaluated to determine if available data can be used, or if new data are necessary, and if so, for what information.
- Identify, from the corporate perspective, potential partners to collaborate with in preparing the CHNA.
- If the CHNA is a collaborative venture, be sure that the hospital's

role is clear, both to those within the hospital and those representing other community stakeholders.

- Allocate appropriate resources for developing the CHNA and the CHIP.
- Determine how and at what level of detail the CHIP will be made public.

- Gain approval of the CHIP from the executive leadership and the hospital board before making it public.
- Read and approve Part VI of Form 990 Schedule H before it is submitted to the IRS.

CHAPTER 5

ACA Integration Initiatives That Promote Collaboration

O ther elements of the Patient Protection and Affordable Care Act (ACA) have implications for partnerships between hospitals and healthcare systems and community organizations. Whereas community health needs assessments (CHNAs) and community health implementation plans (CHIPs) focus on hospital–community coordination at the population level, several aspects of the ACA deal with collaboration between hospitals and other organizations in serving the community primarily for prevention or clinical care at the individual level. The majority of these initiatives address the financing of care, and they focus on Medicare and Medicaid patients—two groups that the hospital might ordinarily seek to minimize because of poor payment.

Most of the ACA initiatives are being tested through demonstrations managed by the Centers for Medicare & Medicaid Services' (CMS) Innovation Center (CMS 2012). Consensus on the definitive direction for any of these initiatives has not yet emerged, and universal regulations are not likely to be enacted for several years while the innovative programs are tested. Moreover, how the ACA evolves over time remains to be determined. However, to the extent that the programs promoted by the ACA deal with the integration of clinical care across settings and over time, strive for high quality with lower costs, and emphasize prevention and the management of chronic illness, these integration initiatives are worthwhile long-term efforts that could well be sustained regardless of federal laws and regulations.

This chapter highlights the ACA provisions that have potential implications for hospital organizational arrangements with other community entities, then it delineates principles of collaboration relevant to multi-entity coordinated clinical care. Regardless of the outcome of the demonstrations or subsequent modifications of the law, hospitals can examine the potential to improve their internal operations by working with external entities more effectively. The lessons learned will have valuable applications for the future.

ACA PROGRAMS

This book makes no pretense of capturing all of the ACA provisions that potentially affect hospitals. It does not address changes in payment mechanisms, quality, or access. However, this section, summarized in Exhibit 5.1, identifies ACA initiatives of particular relevance to the theme of this book: opportunities for hospitals to collaborate with community entities and the organizational processes and structures that facilitate such collaboration. To the extent that ACA initiatives are tested, modified, and eventually incorporated into Medicare or Medicaid conditions of participation or payment mechanisms, the hospitals that have willingly engaged in efforts to achieve successful integration will be ahead of their competitors in market domination, financial stability, and patient and community loyalty. (Further details of the ACA initiatives can be found on the CMS website for the Innovation Center at innovations.cms.gov.)

Partnership for Patients. This umbrella term covers a variety of initiatives. CMS (2012) describes

EXHIBIT 5.1 CMS Innovation Initiatives, 2012

Partnerships for Patients

Community-Based Care Transitions

Accountable Care Organizations

Bundled Payments for Care Improvement

Reduce Avoidable Hospitalizations Among Nursing Facility Residents

Independence at Home

Comprehensive Primary Care

Federally Qualified Health Center Advanced Primary Care Practice

Multipayer Advanced Primary Care Practice Demonstration (medical homes)

Medicaid Incentives Program for the Prevention of Chronic Diseases

SOURCES: CMS (2012, 2011).

it as "a nationwide public–private partnership that aims to reduce [preventable] errors in hospitals by 40 percent and reduce hospital readmissions by 20 percent." By partnering with community-based and institutional long-term care providers as well as patients and families, hospitals can employ a variety of tested techniques to reduce readmissions.

Community-Based Care Transitions Program. Hospitals contract with community-based organizations (CBOs) to coordinate support service upon patient discharge. These part-

nerships help improve the transitions of high-risk Medicare patients from the hospital to other care settings, improve quality of care, reduce readmissions, and document measurable savings to Medicare. Criteria for CBOs are specified by CMS (2012): "Interested CBOs must provide care transition services across the continuum of care and have formal relationships with acute care hospitals and other providers along the continuum of care. An interested CBO must be physically located in the community it proposes to serve, must be a legal entity that can accept payment for services, and have a governing body with representation from multiple healthcare stakeholders including consumers. . . . CBOs will be paid an all-inclusive rate per eligible discharge based on the cost of care transition services provided at the patient level and of implementing systemic changes at the hospital and community levels."

Accountable Care Organizations (ACOs). Provider organizations accept the financial risk for improving quality—including more efficient care coordination—and lowering costs for all of their Medicare patients. CMS (2012) defines ACOs as "groups of doctors, hospitals, and other healthcare providers, who come together voluntarily to give coordinated high-quality care to the Medicare patients they serve. Coordinated care helps ensure that patients, especially the chronically ill, get the right care at the right time, with the goal of avoiding unnecessary duplication of services and preventing medical errors." Several ACO models have been developed, with hospitals, medical groups, and payment mechanisms at the heart of most of them. Other community providers and support organizations are often involved as well. ACOs are one of several CMS initiatives to

which the concept of the patient-centered medical home applies.

Bundled Payments for Care Improvement. This initiative tests several methods for bundling payment for all services rendered to patients during a single episode of care. For the hospital to succeed at bundled payment, relationships between acute and post-acute providers must be efficient and effective at producing high-quality care outcomes. The goal for this initiative is to develop ways to align the financial incentives for hospitals, physicians, and post-acute payers to improve coordination of care and thereby improve quality with lower costs.

Reduce Avoidable Hospitalizations Among Nursing Facility Residents. This initiative supports organizations that partner with nursing facilities to implement evidence-based interventions to both improve care and lower costs. The initiative focuses on long-stay nursing facility residents who are enrolled in Medicare and Medicaid. As evident in the name, the goal is to reduce avoidable inpatient hospitalizations. Hospitals can partner with nursing facilities to share evidence-based practices, staff expertise, medical records, and other techniques that benefit both the hospital and the nursing facility in preventing unnecessary hospital admissions.

Independence at Home Demonstration. This demonstration supplements standard benefits by "providing chronically ill patients with a complete range of primary care services in the home setting. Medical practices led by physicians or nurse practitioners will provide primary care home visits tailored to the needs of beneficiaries with multiple chronic conditions and functional limitations" (CMS 2012). The initiative "will test whether home-based care can reduce the need for hospitalization, improve patient and caregiver satisfaction, and lead to better health and lower costs to Medicare" (CMS 2012). Hospitals, as well as hospital-sponsored medical groups, have been among those awarded grants to test this care-at-home model.

Comprehensive Primary Care. This initiative supports clinicians in managing and coordinating comprehensive care for their patients, particularly those with serious or chronic diseases. Comprehensive Primary Care "supports collaboration between public and private payers and primary care practices that agree to give patients 24-hour access to care, create personalized care plans, and coordinate with other providers

to ensure patients get well and stay healthy" (CMS 2012). The concept of a patient-centered medical home applies here. CMS is working with state-sponsored and commercial health insurance plans to offer extra payments to primary care doctors who are better able to coordinate care for their patients. The goal is to improve access to primary care. Hospitals can be involved to the extent that they offer primary care clinics, subsidize clinics in the community, or work with primary care providers to coordinate specialty or emergency services for those patients who have a primary care provider.

Federally Qualified Health Center (FQHC) Advanced Primary Care Practice. This initiative demonstrates how FQHCs can "act as patient-centered medical homes to improve coordination and quality of care to Medicare patients as well as others. This demonstration project. . . will test the effectiveness of doctors and other health professionals working in teams to coordinate and improve care for Medicare patients. . . . Participating FQHCs are expected to achieve Level 3 patient-centered medical home recognition, help patients manage chronic conditions and . . . adopt care coordination practices that are recognized by the National

Committee for Quality Assurance (NCQA)" (CMS 2012). This initiative includes specific use of the *patient-centered medical home* terminology.

For any of these demonstration initiatives to succeed, hospitals must partner with other organizations in the community. Some relationships—such as those with nursing homes and medical groups—will have a long history. Where agreements are new, senior leaders can contribute by giving guidance in selecting community partners, shaping effective contracts to formalize collaboration, and managing a portfolio of relationships.

LESSONS LEARNED ABOUT INTEGRATION

The US healthcare system has a considerable history of constructing integrated systems to provide a continuum of care. The 1980s and 1990s saw a wave of initiatives that brought together hospitals, physicians, long-term care, managed care, and various other stakeholders. Truly integrated systems, such as Kaiser Permanente, have demonstrated cost savings and superior quality. The ACA's contributions include providing financial incentives to promote integration and applying those incentives on an ongoing basis to large

segments of the population through Medicare and Medicaid. The move toward electronic medical records predates the ACA but is an essential foundation for integrated care that has been lacking until recent federal mandates. The combination of electronic medical records and financial incentives to provide comprehensive and quality care may turn out to be the tipping point that moves the United States away from the fragmented care that exists currently. Management lessons have been learned about integration from both successes and aborted efforts (AHA 2012a; Evashwick and Weiss 1987; Evashwick 1997; National Chronic Care Consortium 2001; Shortell et al. 1996; Shortell, Gillies, and Anderson 2000; Weil, Bogue, and Morton 2001; Zuckerman 2010). This wealth of knowledge can be applied to advancing hospital efforts today. Selected recommendations include the following:

- Choose community partners for long-term strategies, not short-term demonstrations. In the rush to be out front in testing new models (and applying for CMS grants), hospitals should be wary of quick marriages. Long-term relationships between organizations are based on shared values, shared vision, compatible cultures, harmonious leadership, and a solid business case for each organization.

• Articulate partnership terms in writing (including formal contracts), especially for partnerships that involve payment arrangements. When arrangements are put into precise words, seeing if all parties can agree is much easier. Clearly articulated purposes can then be translated into measurable goals and objectives in the accompanying business plan, thereby giving all parties objective criteria to assess whether the agreement is working as expected.

• Allow for a mutually agreeable escape clause. Just as with vendor contracts, having a cancellation clause is important. Maintaining positive relationships with the community and community organizations is much easier if the reasons for cancellation are agreed on up front rather than after a program has launched.

• Gain board approval. The board should represent the range of hospital stakeholders, including the community. Relationships should be approved by the board in advance of implementing a new program, especially if the activity or the partnerships might be controversial.

• Allow sufficient time to build infrastructure, especially for community organizations that might not have the magnitude of operational processes and resources as the hospital. Hospitals, medical groups, and managed care companies are typically the largest entities in the healthcare system of any community. Community agencies want to be players in the partnerships but are likely to be well aware of the difference in resource base. Hospitals walk a fine line in sharing responsibility while balancing appropriate resource contribution. There is no right formula, only issues to be considered.

• Assess the status of partners' information management systems—both for patients and for operations. Because of federal government mandates, hospitals and physician groups are well set up to develop electronic medical records. Other providers are less so. If the hospital expects to track patient utilization across settings, monitor outcomes, share revenue and expenses, and achieve efficiencies of operations, the information management systems of its partners will be critical. Evaluating the status of each organization's information management system and allowing for the time and costs of achieving interoperability or other means of data sharing are critical to the long-term success of a collaboration that goes beyond being superficial.

- Consider relationships from the community residents' standpoint. Relationships made with one partner that require patients and families, as well as referring providers, to use a specific provider might meet with resistance if this runs counter to a well-established utilization pattern. Educating patients, families, and providers and explaining the relationships to them are essential to gain acceptance of new providers. Community residents may treasure preferred providers who provide information on quality and cost.

- Expect resistance to change as formal relationships replace informal patterns. As with changes in patients' customary use patterns, changes that require staff to engage with different organizational partners could well be met with resistance and distrust. Providing information and explanation for staff may be necessary to gain their cooperation.

- Educate the hospital staff and the community partners about the processes and procedures for collaborating on patient empowerment and education. Terminology alone can be a barrier to success if the hospital staff use one set of acronyms and a community agency uses another. Legal requirements might vary or simply be implemented differently. Corporate cultures, if not incompatible, could still vary. Even when willing to make a change, frontline staff of all partner entities should be given the attention and education essential to making future operations smooth.

- Consider formal relationships for a given program within the greater context of multiple relationships. As efforts to coordinate care expand, a hospital might find itself involved with more than one communitywide collaborative or internal care coordination program. Senior leadership might be the only place with a broad enough view or span of control to be aware of all that the organization is doing. Competing or conflicting relationships must be sorted out so that the formal initiatives pursued by the hospital are compatible with one another. Need for resources—including the intangible but essential staff commitment—must also be adjudicated at the highest levels of the hospital leadership or board.

ACTIONS FOR HEALTHCARE EXECUTIVES

- Assign someone at a senior level to monitor the successes (and failures) of current national demonstrations, including lessons learned, and to serve as the planning and organizational liaison with new community-based programs.
- Approach partnerships with community organizations with the same business rigor as the hospital would a merger or acquisition.
- Maintain transparency with the board and close communication with internal and external stakeholders. Both are vital for long-term success even though solidifying the terms of an agreement might require discretion and confidentiality.
- Monitor the actions of competitors and collaborators to assess relationships that might affect the hospital's market.
- Keep the hospital's mission and community in the forefront while positioning the hospital for eventual changes. The ultimate goal of the CMS innovation demonstrations is to test new ways to control the costs and improve quality and access to Medicare and Medicaid.

CHAPTER 6

Action Plan for Hospitals: Internal Focus

T his chapter focuses on what the hospital should do internally to implement a strong infrastructure for maximizing involvement with the community. Three major themes have emerged from hospitals' recent activities with regard to their communities:

1. The hospital's historic relationships with the community that have been assumed now need to be reinforced with vigor and perhaps expanded.
2. Community expectations, accompanied by legal mandates, will continue to evolve, and hospitals must anticipate, create infrastructure for, and lead rather than merely react to these changes.

3. Data are key: Activities with the community must be built on evidence-based practices, justified as priorities, and evaluated with objective measures of results.

Hospitals and health systems that understand these themes have positioned themselves well. Hospitals that have ignored the realities of community involvement have paid the price of challenges to their tax exemption, financial penalties, negative publicity, and lack of community support. One need only search stories in the *Wall Street Journal* to confirm the repercussions of failing to recognize the new stance that hospitals must assume with their communities.

MANAGEMENT ACTIONS

Specific actions by senior leadership are necessary to bolster or promote interactions that can be undertaken and even led by a variety of units within the hospitals. Weil, Bogue, and Morton (2001) noted successful principles of community engagement in their study of model hospital–community dyads. The Advancing the State of the Art in Community Benefit project analyzed community benefit (CB) programs at 70 sites

and produced a list of management practices essential to success (Public Health Institute 2004). Current award programs, such as the American Hospital Association's Foster G. McGaw Prize for Excellence in Community Service and Jackson Healthcare's National Hospital Charitable Service Awards, recognize the importance of management leadership (AHA 2012b; Jackson Healthcare 2013).

Despite being grounded in basic good management practices, many hospitals have not infused their community activities with the rigor that they apply to other aspects of healthcare operations. One study found that only 14 percent of hospitals and 43 percent of systems had assigned oversight for CB activities to a specific standing committee (Prybil et al. 2012). Furthermore, in only 64 percent of healthcare systems had the board adopted a formal, written statement that defines the overall goals and guidelines for the system's CB program (Prybil et al. 2012).

Exhibit 6.1 contains fundamental actions, structures, and processes that hospital executive leaders can take to ensure optimal relationships are developed and maintained with the community. These assume that community health needs, community representatives, and community

> **EXHIBIT 6.1 C-Suite Checklist for Successful Community Engagement**
>
> - Commitment of the board to community involvement
> - Community engagement linked to strategic business directions
> - Composition of board or separate advisory committee to get input from the community
> - Community benefit plan approved by board; possibly separate CB subcommittee
> - C-suite and hospitalwide commitment and accountability to community engagement
> - Senior executive for community affairs as member of the C-suite team
> - Adequate budget for community activities
> - Comprehensive identification of community engagement activities
> - Financial accounting of costs/benefits of community engagement activities
> - Outcome measures linked to improved community health
> - Operations following principles of patient and community respect
> - Staff aware of and engaged in community health improvement
> - Transparent and frequent communications with external and internal stakeholders
> - Goals and objectives of strategic plan include measures of community health improvement

leaders are identified, as described in previous chapters, and incorporated into the fabric of hospital activities. Management actions are at risk of failing if taken in a vacuum, regardless of their good intent.

These actions fall into the general categories of governance, infrastructure, operations, collaboration, and measurement. Each can be struc-

tured to maximize successful relationships with the community.

Governance. The board must be aware of legal mandates and the hospital's activities as they relate to CB, community health needs assessments (CHNAs), and community health implementation plans (CHIPs) as well as system integration initiatives. The CHNA and CHIP should be brought to the board, or at minimum a governing committee, for approval. Schedule H should also be shared annually with the board. System integration projects, even if done under a separate legal entity, should be done with board knowledge and approval.

Governing boards typically include leaders of the community and potential donors. The board composition should also incorporate the viewpoints of the many groups served by the hospital. This might mean allocating seats on the board for community members, but other mechanisms can be used as well to ensure that the board has the broad perspective of the hospital's community. Orientation and education of the board, regular term limits, nominating processes, and level of approval should be examined to ensure they are suitable for the current demands on the hospital to be accountable to its community.

Infrastructure. Long gone are the days when community outreach could be done by the marketing department or mission staff. As recommended elsewhere in the book, community outreach should be a senior-level position included among the hospital's executive leadership. The American College of Healthcare

Executives has a policy statement on "Healthcare Executives' Responsibility to Their Communities" (2011), included in this book's appendix. To count under IRS requirements, CB operations must be distinct from other activities, although CB might be included in a department or unit that also assumes other functions, such as outreach, public relations, or community education. Resources should be allocated to CB in such a way that they can be used effectively and itemized as expenses recognized by the IRS as pertaining to CB, as described in Chapter 3. A separate budget is a good start.

An inventory of which departments and individuals are working in what ways with which community agencies can also be useful, if this is not already done or widely known. Exhibit 6.2 shows a simple inventory format. In this example, pediatrics is engaged in a program that one might typically think would emanate from ob-gyn, thus showing the value of asking the question, "Who is doing what with whom?" The answers might not be obvious. The IRS Schedule H worksheets can be used to gather even more detail about internal relationships, but they are completed retroactively rather than as a snapshot in time.

EXHIBIT 6.2 Inventory of Community Involvement

Department	Community Organizations Involved	Name/Type of Project	Time Frame	Outcome Goals
Pediatrics	Best Babies	Prenatal care for pregnant teens	Grant 2010–2013	Fewer low-birthweight babies (decrease of 10% each year)
Cancer Center	American Cancer Society (local branch), more than 50 community organizations included in online database	Resource center, physical office, and online referral system	Ongoing	Patients linked with resources and support groups (100% of patient inquiries responded to; 90% satisfaction rate)

Operations. Chapter 3 discusses the breadth of hospital activities that might be relevant to CB. New procedures may be useful to capture the data describing these activities with the level of precision required for formal reporting. Hospitals that have created or purchased information management systems, such as the Community Benefit Inventory for Social Accountability (CBISA), are aware of the training that is essential to educate staff about what and how to report. Similarly, new processes may be instituted, such as the way community health needs will be prioritized once a CHNA is prepared, the way activities gain approval for implementation and funding if they must relate to the CHNA, or the way transfer arrangements with community providers have changed. Given all the units and individuals involved in working with the community, the hospital might need to conduct its own internal assessment of activities and relationships before making any decisions about what to report and how to manage reporting, let alone how to guide interactions.

Beyond just the units engaged directly in activities related to CB or integration projects, community engagement should become the culture of the hospital. One initiative is to include community service in annual performance expectations and reviews, which might then require changes to procedures, processes, data collection, and expectations pertaining to human resource management. Changing over the entire hospital to a community orientation is not easy or done overnight; rather, it is done systematically and over time.

Collaboration. *Whom* the hospital partners with and *how* remain two questions central to the concept of community engagement. Recalling the myriad external forces that are prompting community engagement (Exhibit 1.2), the hospital must prioritize which organizations and segments of the community warrant priority attention in any given year. The hospital's strategic plan will offer some guidance, as will the CHNA and the resulting CHIP. Personal relationships will no doubt also continue to influence institutional relationships. Nonetheless, the key to sustainable partnerships is forming them thoughtfully and with purpose. Shared vision and common goals form the basis for active collaboration. Respect, transparency, communication, measurement, collective celebration—all should be built into

the culture of the hospital's operations involving community organizations. Segments of the community that are not represented by formal organizations should also be reached out to, whether through focus groups, key informant interviews, or other grassroots techniques.

Measurement. An evidence-based approach to working on community health issues is feasible and desirable. As noted in Chapter 2, the science of public health has advanced to make available many valid measures that can be employed to study and evaluate hospital activities. Public health informatics has become a distinct field of information management (AMIA 2012). Whether reporting to the board, the IRS, or the community, results reinforced by data and decisions driven by data can be expected to be the norm for the future. Databases, reporting systems, technical expertise among the IT staff—the hospital must treat data related to community programming with the same rigor with which it treats data related to service utilization and clinical care.

MODELS

The AHA awards the Foster G. McGaw Prize for Excellence in Community Service annually. The winners of this award "demonstrate a passion and continuous commitment to making their communities healthier and more vital" according to the following criteria (AHA 2012b):

- **Leadership.** The health delivery organization takes a proactive role in establishing the web of relationships needed to address the community's health and social issues and to improve the community's well-being.
- **Commitment.** Individuals and departments throughout the health delivery organization, including governance, administration, and patient care, are involved on an ongoing basis in the organization's community service plan and/or initiatives.
- **Partnerships.** The health delivery organization has alliances with the community, including physicians, other health-related organizations, businesses, and government, to identify and meet community health needs.
- **Breadth and depth of initiatives.** The organization's community service initiatives: (a) exceed the provision of just acute medical and health care services; (b) address major health-related issues

in the community; (c) constitute a significant and sustainable ongoing effort by the health delivery organization; and (d) demonstrate an impact on the community's health status and/or quality of life.
- **Community involvement.** There is a high level of community response to, acceptance of, and participation in the health delivery organization's community service initiatives.

The list of awardees and additional information can be found at www.aha.org/about/awards/foster/winners.shtml.

The AHA launched an initiative in 2005 called Community Connections. Over the ensuing years, Community Connections has compiled numerous examples of how hospitals work with communities. These case examples, reported annually, are available at www.caringforcommunities.org/caringforcommunities/hospitalsaction/caseexamples.html.

CAVEATS

Community engagement, community benefit, and CHNA are overlapping activities but distinct management tasks. Moreover, how "the community" is defined may not be the same for various hospital initiatives. The ideal approach to working with and for the community might be more of a Rubik's cube than a jigsaw puzzle. In trying to promote logical, evidence-based activities, senior executives should accept that communities and health systems are complex, and interactions might be less than optimal. The long-term vision with the shared goal of optimizing community health status could help smooth rough times along the way.

CEOs are the chief decision makers for a reason. If a physician, community representative, or staff member makes a good enough case for activities or resources, the CEO must be able to exercise the authority to choose actions that are in the best interest of the hospital. Keeping the board apprised of decisions related to community interactions will protect the hospital from the perception of failing to uphold commitments to the community.

ACTIONS FOR HEALTHCARE EXECUTIVES

- Include a goal and measurable objectives related to the community in the hospital's strategic plan.
- Educate the governing board about community initiatives; create one or more ways that the board is informed about and approves hospital activities with the community.
- Analyze the way in which community relationships are conducted internally by the hospital staff and leaders.
- Revamp management structure, processes, and resource allocation to reflect the community engagement imperative.
- Include the position responsible for community activities in the senior leadership of the hospital and health system.
- Incorporate measures related to community engagement into institutional and individual performance assessment, potentially accompanied by thresholds or rewards.
- Recognize individual staff members and units for collaborating with the community.

CHAPTER 7

Action Plan for Hospitals: External Focus

In addition to organizing internal efforts and providing sufficient resources, hospitals must revisit how they are engaged with the community. In past eras, the hospital CEO would be a member of the local Lions Club or Rotary, and that constituted community engagement. Times have changed. Chapter 6 recommends that the hospital keep an inventory of what units are working with which community organizations. Chapter 4 describes how the hospital can collaborate with other organizations on the community health needs assessment (CHNA). These two actions provide vital information about community leaders and existing relationships, which can then be incorporated into a deliberate, strategic approach to engagement with community organizations and individuals representing key stakeholder groups.

Many techniques for involvement with the community are well tested. Engagement requires interaction—the hospital must ask, but also listen; invite, but also offer. The community health implementation plan (CHIP) discussed in Chapter 4 is an opportunity to demonstrate concrete ways that the hospital can work with community organizations on concerns that affect the local population. The hospital has ways to reach out to make its presence known, to bring community members into the organization, or to collaborate. The extent of hospital involvement with community organizations will depend in part on the size and resources of the hospital; on its assets, needs, and goals; and on the size of the community. Methods for involvement include the following:

- Advisory boards of community representatives
- Hospital leaders or program directors as members of boards or committees of community organizations
- Community representatives as members of the hospital's board
- Periodic key informant interviews as part of the overall CHNA process or in conjunction with specific, targeted programs

- Surveys of community members to ask opinions about the hospital or certain programs (different from needs assessment surveys)
- Feedback from patients and community members coming to the hospital in conjunction with care needs (such as patient satisfaction surveys)
- Focus groups of critical stakeholders, particularly regarding specific programs
- Awards programs whereby the hospital recognizes individuals or organizations that contribute to the health of the community
- Scholarships for students to attend educational programs
- Outreach to attract volunteers or auxiliary members from typically underrepresented segments of the community
- Leadership and/or financial support for projects to improve community health status, based on the findings of the CHNA
- Cosponsored community outreach events
- Application by the hospital and community partners for joint grants or for state or national recognition awards

Many relationships will develop in the course of doing business or in response to requests. The CHNA offers a means for seeking input from a wide array of community leaders and lay members. Integration projects, as described in Chapter 5, may be highly focused yet include a distinct set of community agencies. In general, a strategic analysis of community relationships, a plan for engagement, and periodic review move community relationships from random activities initiated by individuals to corporate functions that are sustained over time.

COMMUNITY ASSET ANALYSIS

CHNAs often include a component referred to as the "community asset analysis." This analysis lists health-related resources in the community and provides a critical evaluation of each on key criteria. *Health-related* can be broadly defined to include organizations that focus on factors that affect health indirectly as well as directly. Exhibit 7.1 gives a sample list of the broad categories of organizations that might be included. In this example, a worksheet is used to profile each organization, then the worksheets are rolled up into the summary table. The evaluation

criteria or profile elements should include publicly available information that affects the organization's ability to contribute to the health of the community. Target audience, number of staff, annual operating budget, source of funds, number of people served annually, and communication vehicles are all possible data elements. A federally funded program of promising practices in maternal and child health needs assessments recommends evaluating agencies on the basis of characteristics of accessibility, quality, and affordability (HRSA 2004). The measure of quality can be taken from third-party sources, such as the Nursing Home Compare website (www.medicare.gov/NursingHomeCompare/) or the National Committee for Quality Assurance Health Plan Report Card (CMS 2013; NCQA 2012).

From the hospital's perspective, these organizations can be evaluated for opportunities to reach out for hospital leaders and staff to participate in the organization's activities; to pull in and engage community members in hospital activities; or to collaborate in activities ranging from program planning to service delivery integration (see Exhibit 7.2).

EXHIBIT 7.1 Sample Community Asset Analysis Framework

Category	Target Audience # Services/Year	# Staff	Annual Budget	Communications and Media	Quality Indicators
Health Service Providers					
Home Health, Inc.	_____	_____	_____	_____	_____
Home Support	_____	_____	_____	_____	_____
SNF, Inc.	_____	_____	_____	_____	_____
Mental Health	_____	_____	_____	_____	_____
Health Promotion and Education					
American Diabetes Assn.	_____	_____	_____	_____	_____
American Heart Assn.	_____	_____	_____	_____	_____
Alzheimer's Assn.	_____	_____	_____	_____	_____
Multiservice Organizations					
United Way	_____	_____	_____	_____	_____
Catholic Charities	_____	_____	_____	_____	_____
Jewish Family Services	_____	_____	_____	_____	_____
Local public health dept.	_____	_____	_____	_____	_____
Specialty Subgroups					
Asian-Pacific Coalition	_____	_____	_____	_____	_____
Latino Caucus	_____	_____	_____	_____	_____
Well-Babies!	_____	_____	_____	_____	_____

EXHIBIT 7.2 Opportunities for Engagement

Category	Reach Out	Pull In	Collaborate
Health Service Providers			
Home Health, Inc.			
FQHC Clinic			
SNF, Inc.			
Mental Health			
Health Promotion and Education			
American Diabetes Assn.			
American Heart Assn.			
Alzheimer's Assn.			
Multiservice Organizations			
United Way			
Catholic Charities			
Jewish Family Services			
Local public health dept.			
Specialty Subgroups			
Asian-Pacific Coalition			
Latino Caucus			
Well-Babies!			

ASSESSING HOSPITAL INVOLVEMENT

How structured a hospital should be in orchestrating relationships with the community depends at least in part on the resources of the hospital, its history, and its strategic directions. In a large hospital, just identifying all of the relationships that exist could be an exercise requiring a multidimensional spreadsheet. Once the hospital has goals and objectives pertaining to the community as one element of the hospital's strategic plan, executive leadership should consider:

- relationships with key community organizations that are strategically essential (for example, if the hospital is engaged in creating an accountable care organization);
- how community involvement is promoted to staff;
- if and how community involvement is measured in staff performance reporting; and
- what method(s) will be used to evaluate and realign relationships with the community on an ongoing basis.

Some organizations ask staff to report on an annual basis those organizations with which they are involved informally as well as formally and to keep track of the number of community service hours they volunteer each year. Exhibit 7.3 gives an example of a hospital that started with a systematic approach to being involved with organizations in its community and what happened over time. This example is an extension of the exercise in Exhibit 6.2, overlaying what organizations staff are affiliated

---

EXHIBIT 7.3 Evolution of Community Participation

A hospital's community health department members had spread their community service efforts deliberately so that they had representatives in a number of organizations that provided health and support services to the community. Through personal relationships, department members had been invited to participate in community organizations in a variety of ways.

Over time, department members had changed and community organizations had sprung up, merged, or ceased to operate. The department conducted a preliminary analysis of its representation in the community by listing key organizations serving the community and the level of involvement of department members with each organization. They found that the breadth of their involvement with community agencies had narrowed considerably, replaced by concentration in a few organizations. For example, a senior department member who had been on the board of the local branch of United Way retired, leaving no representative interacting with United Way. In contrast, what had been one member on the board of the local Diabetes Coalition had become two board members and two additional committee chairs. The committees' chairs were recruiting other hospital staff to their activities, resulting in a considerable presence by the hospital in Diabetes Coalition fun runs, screenings, and health education, among other ongoing and occasional events.

Instead of a broad presence, the community outreach had evolved to become consolidated, leaving many community organizations with no representation or regular liaison with the hospital. This assessment, relatively simple to conduct, revealed the opportunity to improve communication and presence between the hospital and the community.

---

with and those organizations desired for affiliation.

This systematic approach might be perceived by some hospitals as too artificial. However, a careful examination of the existing and missed opportunities can help the hospital shape a community outreach plan with direction and details consistent with its methods of operation. Ignoring community engagement results in random efforts by individuals that can be difficult to quantify and harder to value strategically. With the rollout of the Patient Protection and Affordable Care Act (ACA), hospitals will have opportunities to engage in a variety of community-oriented activities at different times as programs and objectives change. Exhibit 7.4 describes the evolution of a collaborative partnership among hospitals and other health organizations that started with a CHNA conducted unilaterally by one hospital and grew into a communitywide collaborative venture.

ACTIONS FOR HEALTHCARE EXECUTIVES

- Identify community organizations and groups that are important for the hospital.

- Assess community asset strengths and weaknesses.
- Identify and assess existing relationships with community organizations.
- Develop a strategic community engagement plan, involving all relevant units of the hospital, to establish communication and collaboration with organizations critical to community health.
- Communicate to employees and affiliates the value of being involved with other organizations in the community.
- Offer ways for community members to participate in hospital activities.
- Establish mechanisms for regularly publicizing and giving visibility to leadership and staff contributions to community organizations.
- Ensure the key community stakeholder groups are represented on the board.
- Establish mechanisms beyond periodic CHNAs and patient satisfaction surveys for seeking community input and feedback on hospital activities.

EXHIBIT 7.4 Evolution of a Community Coalition

Children's National Medical Center (Children's National) in Washington, DC, exemplifies how hospitals can take a grassroots approach to reach out to the community and implement activities through a coalition of community organizations.

Through its Child Health Advocacy Institute (CHAI), Children's National initiated a community health needs assessment (CHNA) in 2009 to examine the health status of the district's youth. The findings showed that the greatest needs were problems that the hospital could not tackle unilaterally. In the spirit of collaboration, Children's National formalized a partnership with the District of Columbia Department of Health and the DC Primary Care Association, an advocacy organization dedicated to strengthening primary care services.

Over a period of 15 months in 2010 and 2011, the partners sponsored four facilitated citywide forums to gather grassroots input from 100 people representing more than 40 community organizations. Through this approach, the partners and community-based organizations created an environment of transparency and accountability in tracking and reporting.

The impact of lessons learned, the Patient Protection and Affordable Care Act, and economic efficiencies catapulted this partnership to expand beyond pediatrics to the entire life cycle. The DC Healthy Communities Collaborative (DCHCC) was created with hospitals and federally qualified health centers in the District of Columbia. Simultaneously, CHAI partnered with the Clinical and Translational Science Institute at Children's National (CTSI-CN), a partnership of Children's National and the George Washington University, and the Georgetown-Howard Universities Center for Clinical and Translational Science. This partnership was awarded a $500,000 grant under the CTSI-CN to develop a novel community-driven, interactive, web-based portal that provides actionable and timely health information to DC communities and promotes collaboration among clinical and translational science awards researchers and community-based organizations.

The DCHCC will use this web portal, DC Health Matters, for information sharing with the community in a bidirectional manner. The portal allows the communities of the District of Columbia and the DCHCC to actively and collectively participate in the planning and implementation of community health improvement as consumers and providers to realize the ultimate vision of "One DC for All." The coalition emphasizes the importance of working with many health and related organizations to accomplish evident and sustainable change throughout the District of Columbia.

CHAPTER **8**

Communication

C ommunicating with the community is essential if all of the other actions taken by the hospital are to be recognized and appreciated for their impact on the health of the local population. Moreover, the Internal Revenue Service (IRS) and the Patient Protection and Affordable Care Act (ACA) promote access to health services by requiring the hospitals to advertise their financial policies and community benefit (CB) activities. Most hospitals aggressively publicize their acute care and physician-related services. A multimedia communications strategy is also now warranted for CB and other community-oriented programs. The hospital's marketing or public relations department should be actively engaged to develop a sophisticated communications initiative to reach internal and external audiences.

MARKETING 101

Marketing can be defined as "letting your customers know that you have exactly the product they want, delivered in the way they want it, at the price they are willing to pay." It is also defined as an "exchange" (Berkowitz 2011). With regard to CB and ACA compliance, the hospital must let its customers—the community as well as patients and their families—know that it is providing a valuable service in exchange for tax exemption; in other words, the benefits to the community are worth the price the community is willing to pay: a waiver of taxes.

Jackson Healthcare, the founder of the National Hospital Charitable Service Awards, has developed a step-by-step guide titled *Leveraging Your Story* to help hospitals explain not only what they are doing with the community but also how those activities result in a positive "return on investment," measured in terms of dollars and improved community health status (Jackson Healthcare 2012).

ACA AND IRS MANDATES AND RATIONALE

The ACA requires hospitals to make available the community health needs assessment (see Chapter 4) in order to maintain tax-exempt status (IRS 2012a). No explicit criteria have yet been laid out for CB reports, except that the CB report must be posted on the Internet and the URL provided to the IRS as part of reporting on Schedule H.

In an effort to ensure transparency with regard to access to services, the ACA requires hospitals to publicize their financial assistance policies and collection policies in specific ways. Under IRS (501)(r) Sections 4–6, hospitals must

- Develop written financial assistance policies (FAPs).
- Have the policies approved by an authorized body (e.g., governing board, committee).
- Provide a plain-language summary of the FAPs.
- Translate the FAPs into any language that is used by 10 percent of the service population.
- Include an application form and instructions that are also translated into languages used by 10 percent or more of the service population.
- Publicize the FAPs, application form, and other related documents as follows:
  – On the hospital website

- In print, available at the hospital; through the mail, by request; and through public displays in the hospital
- To the community (with the exact approach determined by the hospital)

From a strategic perspective, the rationale for publicizing the hospital's activities with the community is not just to meet a legal requirement; it is to engender a positive, long-term relationship with the community. Based on the (negative) experiences of hospitals that have had legal challenges to their tax-exempt status, union strikes or threats thereof, or community protests over potential mergers or acquisitions, the hospital's image in the community and with related community leaders can be significant in enabling or inhibiting strategic business decisions. Regular and honest communications lay a foundation for solid relationships.

TELLING THE STORY

Hospital associations, masters of advocacy, have long encouraged hospitals to tell their story to the community (CHA 2012c; HFMA 2007; VHA 2000). For the lay community, human interest stories, carefully selected pictures, and charts are effective. For boards and community leaders, data and performance trends can elevate the sophistication of the story and demonstrate the underlying management philosophy.

Gautam, Mayer, and Adons (2011) analyzed the CB reports posted on the websites of 100 top-performing hospitals. They found that the less concrete information the hospital had to present, the more generic pictures and white space were included in the report. At the other extreme, a few hospitals posted the text of the technical report prepared according to IRS Schedule H elements, using terms and categories with technical definitions but not ones resonating with the general public. The expertise of the marketing department was not always employed, resulting in reports lacking the consistency of image and readability of other hospital communications prepared for dissemination to external stakeholders.

In short, communicating with the public about CB and hospital policies requires a balance between meeting legal requirements and conveying important information that the target audiences can understand. The hospital should bring the same level of sophistication to the content and format of these messages that it brings to other hospital communications.

MULTIMEDIA COMMUNICATION

The IRS requires that the hospital's annual CB report be posted on the hospital's website. This requires the same attention as that given to all websites and webpages, including the following:

- Format the report to be compatible with the web design.
- Ensure easy access: The link from the main hospital website should be easy to find and navigate.
- Use color and pictures. Page after page of text will meet the legal requirement but will not necessarily be read or convey a positive attitude.
- Use videos with stories to be more compelling to lay readers than text.
- Translate into languages used by community members.
- Design the site to allow accessibility and readability for people with visual or other impairments.

Many hospitals provide a Spanish-language version of the CB report. For communities with large segments speaking another primary language, posting a webpage already translated is preferable to assuming the reader will have a translation function on her computer that preserves the intent and appeal of the English-language version.

Electronic versions of the CB report can be formatted and mined for posting on Facebook, YouTube, and other social media. The hospital should maximize the use of such opportunities to establish its presence among community members who might not ordinarily think of the hospital as a leading community institution. Young adult males, for example, are at high risk of accidents, often uninsured, and avid social media users. Reaching out to them with messages about health insurance, employment opportunities, and financial assistance policies in the event of emergencies could have long-term benefits to the hospital in building a positive image with them for the future generation as well as making them aware in advance of healthcare financing issues.

Being realistic about who uses electronic media and when is equally important. Although financial and bad debt collection policies must be posted on the hospital's website, a person running to the emergency department at the time of an accident is unlikely to be holding his iPhone scanning the website to evaluate the terms of bill payment prior to asking for help. (Moreover, deterring a person from seeking emergency or medically necessary services by discussing billing in advance of treatment is illegal.) Electronic media should be complemented by other forms of communication.

OTHER TYPES OF COMMUNICATION

A hospital can give visibility to its contributions to the community in many ways in addition to electronic media. Indeed, some of the community members most in need of access to healthcare services are arguably those least likely to be reached through electronic media. A strategic communication plan could include the following:

- High-quality print copies of the annual report, heavy with color, pictures, and specific events and individuals
- Stories in print newspapers
- Recognition ads placed in newsletters of other organizations in the community
- Annual community success celebrations

- An annual luncheon for volunteers
- Focus groups of population segments of particular concern
- Community events designed in conjunction with "community-building" activities (according to the Schedule H, Part II definition)

In short, a variety of techniques can be used to give visibility to the hospital's activities with the community. The direct and indirect costs of these efforts, from staff time to write a press release to food costs for a luncheon, must be considered and included in the hospital's budget. If the activities are integral to CB operations, the expenses can be included on Schedule H. If they are marketing expenses, they are not considered CB. As with all other aspects of CB and ACA compliance, the hospital must delineate its alternatives, evaluate the benefits and costs of each, and decide which, among many options, are most appropriate for the hospital's goals and resources.

ACTIONS FOR HEALTHCARE EXECUTIVES

- Understand the new regulations pertaining to developing and making available financial assistance policies (FAPs) to the community.

- Know and comply with IRS requirements to post CHNA and CB reports and make them accessible to the community.
- Involve the marketing or public relations department in creating a strategic plan for communicating about CB programming, financial policies, and overall contribution to the community.
- Follow effective communication and marketing practices in content, format, channeling, and dissemination.
- Communicate frequently with internal and external stakeholders (board, staff, patients, disenfranchised residents, and community organizations, among others) to ultimately shape the hospital's interactions and reaffirm its commitment of service to its community—thereby meeting the challenge of the hospital–community imperative.

APPENDIX

ACHE Policy Statement

HEALTHCARE EXECUTIVES' RESPONSIBILITY TO THEIR COMMUNITIES

July 1989, May 1994, November 1997 (revised), November 2000 (revised), November 2003 (reaffirmed), November 2006 (revised), November 2009 (revised), November 2011 (revised)

Statement of the Issue

The healthcare executive's responsibility to the community is multifaceted. It encompasses a commitment to increasing access to needed care, improving community health status and addressing the societal issues that contribute to poor health and health disparities as well as personally working for the betterment of the community at large. Taking a leadership role in serving the community is the responsibility of all healthcare executives regardless of occupational setting or ownership structure. When providers, individuals and communities work toward common goals, the results can be significant: healthier children, healthier adults, reduced healthcare costs, appropriate use of limited healthcare resources and, ultimately, a healthier community.

Policy Position

The American College of Healthcare Executives (ACHE) believes that all healthcare executives have a professional obligation to serve their communities through support of organizational initiatives and personal involvement in community and civic affairs. In addition, ACHE believes that healthcare executives should take a proactive role in individual and community health improvement efforts. ACHE recognizes that communities vary widely in demographic characteristics, resources, traditions and needs. Therefore, each community may identify different priorities and approaches.

Healthcare executives can lead or participate in community and organizational initiatives through the following actions:

- Actively engage in collaborative efforts with public health and other government agencies, businesses, associations, educational groups, religious organizations, elected officials, financing entities, foundations and others to measure and assess the community's health status, including the most prevalent health problems and concerns, underlying causes, associated risk factors and the diversity of available resources that may be applied to improve the community's well-being.
- Support efforts to eliminate health disparities for vulnerable populations, including reducing barriers to access; increasing the supply of health workers and other resources in underserved communities; systematically collecting race, ethnicity and language preference data of your patients; and training to help healthcare providers deliver culturally competent care.
- Support the dissemination of accurate information about community health status, the services provided and programs available to prevent and treat illness, and patients' responsibility for their own health.

- Participate in efforts to communicate organizational effectiveness in matching healthcare resources with community needs, improved clinical outcomes and community health status, and their organization's volunteerism roles.
- Incorporate community service responsibilities into policies and programs over which they have authority.
- Demonstrate that their commitment to the community is multifaceted and may include support of medical research, training of healthcare professionals, charity care and civic contributions as well as a host of other activities that contribute to the community's well-being beyond that of their own organization.
- Offer health promotion and illness prevention programs to their employees, positively benefiting staff as well as sending an important message to the community.

Healthcare executives can personally demonstrate their commitment to the community through the following actions:

- Embrace a healthy lifestyle. ACHE affiliates should model behavior they are advocating for their employees and the community at large. Appropriate behavior may include exercising regularly, refraining from smoking, adopting a healthy diet, taking steps to reduce stress and getting preventive checkups to address health problems before they become serious.
- Participate in local assessments of community need.
- Be the catalyst for community-based interventions.
- Participate in regional, state and local task forces to resolve health disparities and other community healthcare problems.
- Actively advocate for the community with the public, policymakers and other key stakeholders to define community healthcare priorities so that healthcare resources can be used equitably and effectively.
- Become involved in community service projects, civic organizations and public dialogue on healthcare policy issues affecting the community.
- Share models of successful healthy community projects with others to enhance efforts in other communities.

ACHE urges all healthcare executives to affirm their responsibility to their communities through their professional actions and personal contributions. To further strengthen its position on community responsibility, ACHE requires its affiliates to produce evidence of participation and leadership in healthcare and community/civic affairs to advance within ACHE.

Approved by the Board of Governors of the American College of Healthcare Executives on November 14, 2011.

References

Agency for Healthcare Research and Quality (AHRQ). 2012. "National Quality Measures Clearinghouse." Accessed November 1. www.quality measures.ahrq.gov.

American College of Healthcare Executives (ACHE). 2011. "Healthcare Executives' Responsibility to Their Communities." Accessed December 13, 2012. www.ache.org/policy/Respon.cfm.

American Hospital Association (AHA). 2012a. "Community Connections Project." Accessed December 6. www.caringforcommunities.org.

———. 2012b. "Foster G. McGaw Prize: Call for Entries." Accessed December 13. www.aha.org/about/awards/foster/application.shtml.

American Medical Informatics Association (AMIA). 2012. "Public Health Informatics." Accessed October 24. www.amia.org/programs/working-groups/public-health-informatics.

Association for Community Health Improvement (ACHI). 2012. "Home Page." Accessed October 23. www.communityhlth.org.

———. 2007. "Community Health Assessment Toolkit." Accessed October 24. www.assesstool kit.org.

Barsi, E. 2009. "Community Benefit: Moving Forward with Evidence-Based Policy and Practice." Presentation at the preconference to the Annual Research Meeting of Academy Health, Chicago, June 27.

Berkowitz, E. 2011. *Essentials of Health Care Marketing,* 3rd ed. Sudbury, MA: Jones & Bartlett Learning.

Brownson, R., E. Baker, T. Leet, K. Gillespie, and W. True. 2011. *Evidence-Based Public Health,* 2nd ed. New York: Oxford University Press, Inc.

Catholic Health Association (CHA). 2012a. *Assessing & Addressing Community Health Needs.* St. Louis, MO: Catholic Health Association.

———. 2012b. "Community Benefit." Accessed October 23. www.chausa.org/communitybenefit.

———. 2012c. "Ministry Examples." Accessed December 11. www.chausa.org/Pages/Our_Work/ Community_Benefit/Ministry_Examples/Overview/.

———. 2011. *Assessing & Addressing Community Health Needs.* Published March 1. www.vha .com/AboutVHA/PublicPolicy/CommunityBenefit/Documents/AssessingAddressing CH.pdf.

———. 2008. "Explaining the New Rules for Measuring Community Benefit." *Health Progress* 89 (5): 46–49.

———. 1989. *Social Accountability Budget: A Process for Planning and Reporting Community Service in a Time of Fiscal Constraint.* St. Louis, MO: Catholic Health Association.

Centers for Medicare & Medicaid Services (CMS). 2013. "Nursing Home Compare." Accessed January 23. www.medicare.gov/NursingHomeCompare/.

———. 2012. "CMS Innovation Center." Accessed December 13. www.innovations.cms.gov.

———. 2011. "One Year of Innovation." Accessed November 4, 2012. innovations.cms.gov/Files/ reports/Innovation-Center-Year-One-Summary-document.pdf.

Community Catalyst. 2007. *Health Care Community Benefits: A Compendium of State Laws.* Boston, MA: Community Catalyst.

Comprehensive Health Planning and Public Services Act. 1966. Pub. L. No. 89-749.

Congressional Budget Office (CBO). 2006. *Nonprofit Hospitals and the Provision of Community Benefits.* Washington, DC: Congressional Budget Office.

Evashwick, C. J. 1997. *Seamless Connections.* Chicago: American Hospital Association.

Evashwick, C. J., and E. Barsi. 2012. "Community Connections," in *Futurescan 2012: Healthcare Trends and Implications 2012–2017,* 27–32. Chicago: Health Administration Press.

Evashwick, C. J., and L. Weiss. 1987. *Managing the Continuum of Care.* Rockville, MD: Aspen Publishers.

Fleming, S. 2008. *Managerial Epidemiology,* 2nd ed. Chicago: Health Administration Press.

Frechtling, J. 2007. *Logic Modeling Methods in Program Evaluation.* San Francisco: Jossey-Bass.

Gautam, K., J. Mayer, and B. Adons. 2011. "How Does Your Public Report Stack Up?" *Health Progress* 92 (3): 72–73.

Government Accountability Office (GAO). 2008. *Nonprofit Hospitals: Variation in Standards and Guidance Limits Comparison of How Hospitals Meet Community Benefit Requirements.* GAO-08-880. Published September 1. www.gao.gov/new.items/d08880.pdf.

Healthcare Financial Management Association (HFMA). 2007. *Telling the Community Benefit Story: An HFMA Educational Report.* Accessed January 22, 2013. www.hfma.org/Content.aspx?id = 1141.

———. 2006. "Statement 15: Valuation and Financial Statement Presentation of Charity Care and Bad Debts by Institutional Healthcare Providers." Published December 1. www.hfma.org/Templates/InteriorMaster.aspx?id = 17946.

Healthy Communities Institute. 2012. "Home Page." Accessed November 2. www.healthy communitiesinstitute.com.

Institute of Medicine (IOM). 2011. *For the Public's Health: The Role of Measurement in Action and Accountability.* Washington, DC: The National Academies Press.

———. 2002. *Who Will Keep the Public Healthy? Educating Public Health Professionals for the 21st Century.* Washington, DC: The National Academies Press.

Internal Revenue Service (IRS). 2012a. "Form 990." Accessed December 11. www.irs.gov/form990.

———. 2012b. "Specific Instructions." Accessed December 11. www.irs.gov/instructions/i990sh/ch02.html.

———. 2011. "Notice and Request for Comments Regarding the Community Health Needs Assessment Requirements for Tax-Exempt Hospitals." *Notice 2011.52.* Accessed December 11. www.irs.gov/pub/irs-drop/n-11-52.pdf.

———. 2007. "IRS Releases Interim Report on Tax-Exempt Hospitals and Community Benefit Project." Accessed November 2, 2012. www.irs.gov/uac/IRS-Releases-Interim-Report-on-Tax-Exempt-Hospitals-and-Community-Benefit-Project.

———. 1969. "Revenue Ruling 69-545 1969-2 C.B. 117." Accessed December 11. www.irs.gov/pub/irs-tege/rr69-545.pdf.

Jackson Healthcare. 2013. "Hospital Charitable Service Awards." Accessed January 23. www.jacksonhealthcare.com/give-back.aspx#st_content_1.

———. 2012. *Leveraging Your Story.* Accessed October 24. www.jacksonhealthcare.com/awards/community/resources/ebooks/return-on-invested-giving.aspx.

Lyon Software. 2012. "CBISA for Healthcare." Accessed January 22, 2013. www.lyonsoftware.com/products/cbisa-hc-index.php.

McAlearney, A. 2003. *Population Health Management: Strategies to Improve Outcomes.* Chicago: Health Administration Press.

National Association of County and City Health Officials (NACCHO). 2013. "Toolkit." Accessed January 22. www.naccho.org/toolbox/veritysearch/search.cfm?keywords = Data&p = ALL&st = A LL&jurisdiction = ALL&x = 63&y = 13.

———. 2012. "MAPP Framework." Accessed October 12. www.naccho.org/topics/infrastructure/mapp/framework/index.cfm.

National Chronic Care Consortium. 2001. "Self-Assessment for Systems Integration Tool." Accessed November 16, 2012. www.nccconline.org/SASI/SASi_Objectives.pdf.

National Committee for Quality Assurance (NCQA). 2012. "NCQA's Health Insurance Plan Rankings 2012-2013—Private Plan Details." Accessed November 2. www.ncqa.org/Portals/0/Report%20Cards/Rankings/hpr2012privatedet.pdf.

New York State Department of Health. 2009. "2010–2013 Community Health Assessment Guidance." Accessed December 11, 2012. www.health.ny.gov/statistics/chac/nysguidance.htm.

North Carolina Division of Public Health. 2010. *Community Health Assessment Guide Book.* http://publichealth.nc.gov/lhd/cha/docs/CHA-GuideBookUpdatedDecember15-2011.pdf.

Patient Protection and Affordable Care Act (ACA). 2010. Pub. L. No. 111-148, 125 Stat 119.

Pennsylvania Hospital. 2012. "Mission Statement." Accessed November 26. www.pennmedicine.org/pahosp/about/mission.html.

Prybil, L., S. Levey, R. Killian, D. Fardo, R. Chait, D. Bardach, and W. Roach. 2012. *Governance in Large Nonprofit Health Systems: Current Profile and Emerging Patterns.* Lexington, KY: Commonwealth Center for Governance Studies, Inc.

Public Health Accreditation Board (PHAB). 2012. "Standards and Measures." Accessed August 8. www.phaboard.org/accreditation-process/public-health-department-standards-and-measures/.

Public Health Institute. 2004. *Advancing the State of the Art in Community Benefit: A User's Guide to Excellence and Accountability.* Accessed October 23. www.communityhlth.org/communityhlth/projects/asacb/asacbhome.html.

Seay, J. D., and R. M. Sigmond. 1989. "Community Benefit Standards for Hospitals: Perceptions and Performance." *Frontiers of Health Services Management* 5 (3): 3–39.

Senate Committee on Finance—Minority. 2007. "Tax-Exempt Hospitals: Discussion Draft." Accessed April 1, 2012. www.grassley.senate.gov/releases/2007/07182007.pdf.

Shortell, S., R. Gillies, and D. Anderson. 2000. *Remaking Health Care in America: The Evolution of Organized Delivery Systems*, 2nd ed. San Francisco: Jossey-Bass.

Shortell, S., R. Gillies, D. Anderson, K. Erickson, and J. Mitchell. 1996. *Remaking Health Care in America: Building Organized Delivery Systems,* 1st ed. San Francisco: Jossey-Bass.

Sibley Memorial Hospital. 2012. "About Sibley Memorial Hospital." Accessed November 26. www.sibley.org/general_info/about_sibley_memorial_hospital.aspx.

St. Joseph's Hospital and Medical Center. 2012. "Mission, Vision, and Values." Accessed January 8, 2013. www.stjosephs-phx.org/Who_We_Are/Mission_Vision_And_Values/index.htm

Studer, Q. 2009. *Straight A Leadership: Alignment, Action, Accountability.* Gulf Breeze, FL: Fire Starter Publishing.

Substance Abuse and Mental Health Services Agency (SAMHSA). 2012. "National Registry of Evidence-Based Programs and Practices." Accessed November 29. www.nrepp.samhsa.gov.

University of Pennsylvania Health System. 2012. "The Cornerstone." Accessed November 26. www.uphs.upenn.edu/paharc/timeline/1751/tline3.html.

US Centers for Disease Control and Prevention (CDC). 2013. *Community Assessment for Population Health Improvement: Resource of Frequently Recommended Health Outcomes and Determinants.* Atlanta, GA: Office of Surveillance, Epidemiology, and Laboratory Services.

———. 2012a. "10 Essential Public Health Services." Accessed October 24. www.cdc.gov/nphpsp/essentialServices.html.

———. 2012b. "The Community Guide." Accessed August 6. www.thecommunityguide.org.

———. 2012c. "The Community Guide: Cancer Prevention and Control: Client-Oriented Interventions to Increase Breast, Cervical, and Colorectal Cancer Screening." Accessed January 10, 2013. www.thecommunityguide.org/cancer/screening/client-oriented/index.html.

US Department of Health and Human Services (HHS). 2012. "Healthy People 2020." Accessed August 24. www.healthypeople.gov.

US Department of Health and Human Services Health Resources and Services Administration (HRSA). 2004. "Promising Practices in MCH Needs Assessment: A Guide Based on a National Study." Accessed December 16, 2012. ftp://ftp.hrsa.gov/mchb/naguide.pdf.

VHA, Inc. 2000. *Messages and Strategies for Community-Owned Health Care Organizations: A Guide to Communicating Value.* Accessed December 12, 2012. www.communityhlth.org/communityhlth/files/files_resource/Community%20Benefit/MessagesStrategiesVHA.pdf.

Weil, P., R. Bogue, and R. Morton. 2001. *Achieving Success Through Community Leadership.* Chicago: Health Administration Press.

Zuckerman, A. 2010. *Leading Your Healthcare Organization Through a Merger or Acquisition.* Chicago: Health Administration Press.

About the Author

Connie J. Evashwick, ScD, LFACHE, holds bachelor's and master's degrees from Stanford University and master's and doctoral degrees from the Harvard School of Public Health. She is credentialed in public health (CPH) and association management (CAE) and is a Life Fellow of the American College of Healthcare Executives. Dr. Evashwick has been vice president of long-term care for two major healthcare systems and has authored more than 112 papers and 12 books. Her expertise includes the continuum of care, long-term care delivery systems, and health professions education. More recently she has focused on hospital community benefit and public health systems.